MedStudy®

12th Edition

Internal Medicine Review Core Curriculum

Book 2 of 5

Topics in this volume:

Pulmonary Medicine

Nephrology

Authored by Robert A. Hannaman, MD

MEDSTUDY
1761 South 8th Street, Building H1
Colorado Springs, Colorado 80906
(800) 841-0547

MedStudy®

12th Edition
Internal Medicine Review Core Curriculum

Pulmonary Medicine

Authored by Robert A. Hannaman, MD

Many thanks to

Robert A. Balk, MD
Professor of Medicine
Director, Section of Pulmonary Medicine
Director of Pulmonary and Critical Care
Fellowship Training Program
Rush-Presbyterian-St. Luke's Medical Center
Chicago, Illinois

Pulmonary Medicine Advisor

Pulmonary Medicine

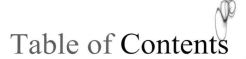

Table of Contents

Pulmonary Medicine

DIAGNOSTIC TESTS

Bronchoalveolar lavage (BAL) is an important pulmonary diagnostic tool. Know Table 3-11 on pg 3-54.

Transbronchial biopsy (TBB) is most useful in diagnosing sarcoidosis and infectious diffuse infiltrative lung diseases. In sarcoidosis, the yield is highest when there are infiltrates on the chest x-ray (90%). It is lowest when there is hilar adenopathy only (70%). Sarcoidosis is also a diagnosis of exclusion; you may see noncaseating granuloma in a number of disease states, such as granulomatous infections and berylliosis.

An open lung biopsy is required to confirm the diagnosis of some causes of idiopathic pulmonary fibrosis (IPF), because IPF is a diagnosis of exclusion and many diseases mimic it (hypersensitivity pneumonitis, eosinophilic granulomatosis, bronchiolitis-obliterans–organizing pneumonia, and lymphangioleiomyomatosis). IPF, by definition, has histologic findings of usual interstitial pneumonitis (UIP). UIP has classic radiological findings also and, about half the time, IPF/UIP can be diagnosed with HRCT. Again, open lung biopsy: think IPF. Usual interstitial pneumonitis (UIP) is diagnosable by a characteristic high-resolution chest CT.

CT scan is used extensively in pulmonary medicine and will also be discussed along with the diseases. High-resolution CT (HRCT—cross sections of 1–2 mm vs. the usual 5–10 mm) is used especially for evaluating airway and parenchymal diseases of the lungs such as bronchiectasis, emphysema, and the interstitial lung diseases—and especially IPF, sarcoidosis, hypersensitivity pneumonitis, Langerhan cell histiocytosis, alveolar proteinosis, and lymphangioleiomyomatosis.

Helical CT is a rapid CT scanning technique that allows increased coverage in a single breath and subsequent, computerized reconstruction of the data into a 3-dimensional image.

Multidetector CT (MDCT) is the next generation of helical CT (previously: single-detector helical CT). It allows 1.2 mm sections during a single held breath. Besides use for the same indications as the HRCT, the MDCT is now often used in place of a V/Q scan when the patient has cardiopulmonary problems that might obscure the results of the V/Q scan.

MRI is useful only in specific cases: When evaluating tumors near adjacent blood vessels or nerves—for determining what is tumor and what is not (e.g., superior sulcus tumors, brachial plexus tumors, mediastinal tumors, tumors near the aorta or heart). CT is still best for lung parenchyma.

Pleural biopsy may be closed or thorascopic.

Pulmonary angiogram is the gold standard for pulmonary embolism diagnosis.

PET scan is useful in differentiating benign vs. malignant pulmonary nodules and infection.

Thoracentesis is covered under pleural effusions.

V/Q scanning is covered under pulmonary embolism.

PFTs are covered below.

RESPIRATORY PHYSIOLOGY
HYPOXEMIA

Note: Acid-Base is covered in depth in the Nephrology section.

Know respiratory physiology well. The information pops up repeatedly on the boards.

Short review:

Atmospheric pressure (P_b): The pressure of the atmosphere varies. At sea level and at 59°F, it is 29.92 inches Hg or 760 mmHg. The medical standard is to use mmHg. Atmospheric pressure decreases as you get further away from the surface of the earth, and also as temperature increases. The component gases of the atmosphere each exerts a consistent partial pressure to the atmospheric pressure. E.g.:

Partial pressure O_2 $= F_iO_2$ x P_b
$= .209 (F_iO_2)$ x 760 mmHg
$= 158.84$ mmHg in the air surrounding us

at sea level at 59°F. This pressure is called the P_iO_2 (inspired). This fraction of 20.9% remains constant as atmospheric pressure decreases with increasing altitude.

The following is the alveolar air equation. It calculates the partial pressure of O_2 in the alveoli.

$$P_AO_2 = [(P_b\text{-}P_{H2O}) \text{ x } F_iO_2] - [P_aCO_2/0.8]$$

This equation looks different from the simpler P_iO_2 equation just discussed. The reason is because the partial pressure of inspired gases changes a little when it gets into the damp alveoli, where O_2-CO_2 exchange occurs. Here, we must account for the additional partial pressure of water vapor P_{H2O} (= 47 mmHg at sea level) and the shifts in concentrations of O_2 and CO_2 in the alveoli. The respiratory quotient (0.8) is the minute production of CO_2 / minute consumption of O_2. This quotient allows us to use the measurable P_aCO_2 (arterial) in the alveolar air equation instead of the P_ACO_2, which we can't readily measure.

So, to get back to the alveolar air equation:
$$P_AO_2 = [(P_b\text{-}P_{H2O}) \text{ x } F_iO_2] - [P_aCO_2/0.8]$$

We see that the F_iO_2 is still multiplied by the P_b but only after its value is decreased to account for the water vapor. The second term will decrease this product by an amount that takes into account the O_2-CO_2 exchange going on in the alveoli.

We'll now go over a few other items, and then go a little more into this!

Other terms:

P_aO_2 = Partial pressure of oxygen in the arteries. Commonly called the "PO2."

P_aCO_2 = Partial pressure of carbon dioxide in the arteries. Commonly called the "PCO2."

S_aO_2 = Oxygen saturation of hemoglobin in the arteries. Also use S_{PaO2} (pulse oximetry).

$S_{\bar{V}}O_2$ = Mixed venous oxygen saturation. Mixed venous blood is in the pulmonary artery.

notes

Hypoxemia has 6 causes:

1) V/Q mismatch: The main cause of hypoxemia in chronic lung diseases—it responds to 100% O_2. It may be due to airspace not being perfused or perfused areas not being ventilated. Examples: Asthma, COPD, alveolar disease, interstitial disease, and pulmonary vascular disease, such as pulmonary hypertension or pulmonary embolism. These diseases respond to oxygen.

2) Right-to-Left shunting: The main cause of hypoxemia in ARDS in which shunting is due to collapse of the alveoli. ARDS does not respond well to 100% O_2; it responds better to positive end-expiratory pressure (PEEP). Discussed more later. Other causes besides alveolar collapse: Intra-alveolar filling (pneumonia, pulmonary edema), intracardiac shunt, and vascular shunt.

3) Hypoventilation: e.g., stopping breathing—always has a high P_aCO_2 associated with the hypoxemia. The A-a gradient ($D_{A-a}O_2$—discussed next) is normal. Think drug overdose.

4) Decreased diffusion: Actually has little causal effect on hypoxemia! It takes a tremendous amount of thickening of the alveolar-capillary interface to decrease diffusion of O_2. Think of the interstitial lung diseases (ILDs) and emphysema, which do improve with supplemental O_2. The CO diffusing capacity (DLCO), therefore, has little clinical value (see below). Low DLCO causes hypoxemia when the DLCO is $\leq$ 30% of predicted and/or with rapid heart rate. With rapid heart rate, the time for diffusion is limited, and decreased O_2 transfer occurs. Increased DLCO is seen with alveolar hemorrhage.

5) High altitudes (low F_iO_2): The A-a gradient ($D_{A-a}O_2$) is normal unless lung disease is present.

6) Low, mixed venous O_2 (P_VO_2): This can decrease the P_aO_2 during resting conditions, secondary to the normal shunt that exists (~ 5%), and will also exaggerate all other causes of low P_aO_2.

So, with the above causes of hypoxemia:

- Supplemental O_2 does not cause significant increase in P_aO_2 with R-to-L shunting or shunt physiology.
- A-a gradient is normal with hypoventilation and high altitudes.

A-a GRADIENT

The alveolar-arterial gradient (A-a gradient) or A-a O_2 ($D_{A-a}O_2$) is the difference between the partial pressure of oxygen in alveoli (A) and that in arterial blood (a):

$$D_{A-a}O_2 = P_AO_2 - P_aO_2$$

The P_AO_2 is relatively consistent in a group of people in a room. The P_aO_2 is what may vary individually with lung problems. It is the difference between these 2 partial pressures that is the key indicator. And again, $D_{A-a}O_2$ is increased in all causes of hypoxemia except hypoventilation and high altitude.

$D_{A-a}O_2$ is 5–15 in healthy young patients. It increases normally with age and abnormally in lung diseases, causing a V/Q

mismatch—i.e., shunt or diffusion abnormality. Note: A patient with a significant pulmonary embolus invariably has an increased $D_{A-a}O_2$ but, if the patient is hyperventilating (which is common), the ABG may show a normal P_aO_2!

As mentioned, $D_{A-a}O_2$ increases with age. 2 rules-of-thumb for determining normal $D_{A-a}O_2$ are:

1) Normal $D_{A-a}O_2 \leq$ 0.3 x Age (years)
or
2) Normal $D_{A-a}O_2 \leq$ (Age/4) + 4

To find the $D_{A-a}O_2$, first determine the partial pressure of O_2 in the alveoli (P_AO_2)—discussed at the beginning of this section.

$$P_AO_2 = [(P_b-P_{H2O}) \times F_iO_2] - [P_aCO_2/0.8]$$

And at standard temperature at sea level:

$$P_AO_2 = [(760-47) \times .209] - [P_aCO_2/0.8]$$

$$P_AO_2 = [149] - [P_aCO_2/0.8]$$
or, to more easily mentally calculate,
$$P_AO_2 = 149 - 1.25(P_aCO_2)$$

So, getting back to the original formula...

$$D_{A-a}O_2 = P_AO_2 - P_aO_2$$
...where the P_aO_2 is obtained from the arterial blood gas.

Or, to more easily calculate it mentally, the formula is shifted around to:

$$D_{A-a}O_2 = 149 - (P_aO_2 + 1.25P_aCO_2)$$

Okay, got this? The P_aCO_2 and the P_aO_2 are read off of the arterial blood gas report. Take a quarter more than the P_aCO_2 and add it to the P_aO_2, then subtract the result from 149. EASY!! Get so you can do this in the blink of an eye, and you might even put some of the pulmonary docs to shame.

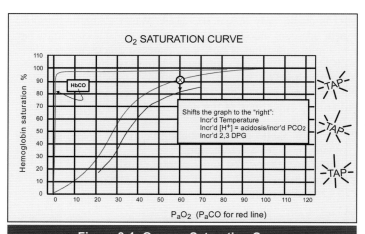

Figure 3-1: Oxygen Saturation Curve

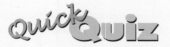
But…but… Yes, good question… What happens at high altitude? What if you live in Colorado Springs, Colorado—at 6500 ft? For each 1000 ft increase in altitude, the atmospheric pressure drops about 25 mmHg. Look at the table in appendix A at the end of this section. At 6,500 ft, the atmospheric pressure is about 596 mmHg—quite a change from sea level! Will this quickie formula work? No! But with a little change for your particular altitude, it will. In the part of the alveolar air equation $[(P_b-P_{H2O}) \times F_iO_2]$, just change the $(760-47) \times .209$ to $(596-37) \times .209 = 117$. Note that the water vapor pressure is proportionately decreased. So in Colorado Springs, we do the same thing—read the P_aCO_2 and the P_aO_2 off of the arterial blood gas report. Take a quarter more than the P_aCO_2 and add it to the P_aO_2, but subtract the result from 117. Calculate it for your altitude.

But…but… Yes, right again. If the patient is on supplemental O_2, just plug the actual F_iO_2 into the equation.

For dropping barometric pressure, see appendix A (pg 3-55).

This increase in altitude can cause quite a drop in P_aO_2. Are you and your patients getting enough oxygen? We'd better discuss oxygen delivery to the tissues.

OXYGEN DELIVERY TO TISSUES

Overview

What is important to the tissues is how much oxygen they receive. This depends on:

I) the amount of oxygen transported to the tissues, and

II) once this oxygen arrives at the tissues, how much is taken up and subsequently utilized by the mitochondria and/or cells.

I) First, we will discuss oxygen transport to the tissues (= DO_2).
DO_2 = Cardiac output x Oxygen content of arterial blood (C_aO_2)
and
$C_aO_2 = (1.34 \times Hgb\ level \times S_aO_2) + .003 x P_aO_2$
(We will ignore the O_2 dissolved in plasma: $.003 \times P_aO_2$).
so
DO_2 = cardiac output x $(1.34 \times Hgb\ level \times S_aO_2)$

Notice in the previous equation, oxygen transported to the tissues depends on 3 factors:
1) Cardiac output
2) Hemoglobin level
3) Hemoglobin saturation (S_aO_2), not P_aO_2! This is why the hemoglobin-oxygen (oxyhemoglobin) dissociation curve (and the use of pulse oximetry) is so important.

These are also the 3 factors you look at when a critically ill patient requires better oxygen delivery. In board questions, you typically are given a critically ill patient with either cardiac output or Hgb level obviously low and S_aO_2, which is 90% with a P_aO_2 of 60 mmHg. The answer is to address the obviously low Hgb or cardiac output—the P_aO_2 is fine because the S_aO_2 is fine!

Oxygen Saturation Curve

The oxyhemoglobin dissociation curve (oxygen saturation curve, Figure 3-1) shows the amount of O_2 saturation of hemoglobin (S_aO_2) for a certain P_aO_2. It is the amount of O_2-saturated Hgb that is important. You can see from the graph that, everything else being normal, a P_aO_2 of 60 mmHg will still result in a S_aO_2 of > 90%.

The actual oxygen saturation of a particular hemoglobin molecule at a particular P_aO_2 is dependent on temperature, erythrocyte 2,3-DPG level, and pH status. The oxyhemoglobin dissociation curve shows the S_aO_2 for a certain P_aO_2—given variations in these 3 factors.

When the graph is shifted to the "right," it reflects a decrease in Hgb affinity for O_2 (so a decreased O_2 uptake by the Hgb). Decreased affinity promotes off-loading of the O_2 to the tissues.

With a shift to the "left" (decreased levels of these same factors), it reflects an increased affinity for O_2 (so an increased S_aO_2 for a particular P_aO_2). High or low levels of serum phosphorus cause an increased or decreased 2,3-DPG.

The blue line on the graph indicates what most people call a "shift to the right," but it is more logical to think of it as a "shift down" in which, for a certain P_aO_2, the S_aO_2 is decreased. On the graph, at a P_aO_2 of 60, the O_2 saturation decreases from 92% to 82%.

Note that the TAP, TAP, TAP on the right of the graph is to remind you of the factors that shift the graph to the right—increased Temp, Acidosis, and Phosphorus (rrright, a tap tap...!)

Carbon monoxide poisoning: If axes of the graph showed P_aCO vs. HgbCO, we would see a tracing (as shown) far to the left. The oxyhemoglobin dissociation curve would be shifted grotesquely to the right/down—showing Hgb O_2 saturation (S_aO_2) only minimally affected by increasing P_aO_2.

Methemoglobin is produced when the iron in the Hgb molecule is oxidized from the ferrous to the ferric form, and the methemoglobin molecule can no longer hold onto O_2 or CO_2—with disastrous results in the tissues. Methemoglobin causes a similar curve shift as CO, in which very high P_aO_2

notes

levels results in low S_aO_2. It may be acquired (drugs) or hereditary. Clinical effects:

- > 25% = perioral and peripheral cyanosis
- 35–40% = fatigue and dyspnea begin
- > 60% = coma, death

Treatment for methemoglobinemia is 100% O_2, remove the source, and methylene blue (which causes rapid reduction of methemoglobin back to hemoglobin). Chronic, hereditary methemoglobinemia is best treated with 1–2 grams daily of ascorbic acid.

Know that the normal oximeter, which measures the absorption of 2 wavelengths of light, is not accurate (and should not be used) when there are significant levels of CO or methemoglobin. A usually-not-readily-available "CO-oximeter" (pronounced co-oximeter) measures 4 wavelengths and distinguishes oxyhemoglobin, deoxygenated Hgb (measures blood gas sample rather than usual calculation of S_aO_2 on ABG), carboxyhemoglobin, and methemoglobin.

II) Okay, we discussed oxygen transport to the tissues. What about actual oxygen release to the tissues? Here again, we look at the oxyhemoglobin dissociation curve. Any factor that shifts the graph to the right/down reflects a decreased affinity between oxygen and hemoglobin and, in the local tissue environment, causes a release of oxygen to the tissues.

E.g., Working muscles: In the area of the capillaries of working muscles, there is an increase of pCO_2 due to normal metabolism → local acidosis → decreased affinity of Hgb for O_2 → release of O_2 to the tissues (Bohr effect).

E.g., RBCs: RBCs produce 2,3-diphosphoglycerate (2,3-DPG) as a byproduct of anaerobic metabolism (all RBC metabolism is anaerobic). The more 2,3-DPG there is, the more O_2 is released from the Hgb for use by the RBCs. Similarly, patients with chronic anemia have increased 2,3-DPG.

E.g., Blood stored > 1 week has a decreased level of 2,3-DPG, and large transfusions of this blood results in a "shift to the left."

When there is systemic acidosis (or high temp or high 2,3-DPG), the decrease in affinity for O_2 by Hgb results in less O_2 picked up by the Hgb in the lung, but also more O_2 released in the tissues. So, although the Hgb O_2 saturation (S_aO_2) is lower for a certain P_aO_2, more of the oxygen carried by the hemoglobin is released to the tissue. The net result is to dampen the effect of low S_aO_2 caused by acidosis, high temp, and high 2,3-DPG. It dampens but does not negate or reverse the effect.

Conditions that shift the graph to the left (alkalosis, low temp, low 2,3-DPG) work similarly, although more O_2 is bound by the Hgb, and less is released to the tissues. Again, it dampens but does not negate the effect.

DLCO

Carbon monoxide diffusing capacity (DLCO) is decreased by anything that interrupts gas-blood O_2 exchange. Not used much...except on Board exams!

Decrease in DLCO implies a loss of effective, capillary-alveolus interface. It is usually due to loss of alveolar-capillary units, as seen in emphysema, interstitial lung disease (diffuse interstitial fibrosis, sarcoidosis, asbestosis), pneumonectomy, and pulmonary vascular problems such as chronic PE or pulmonary hypertension. A decrease is seen with anemia, but usually the DLCO is reported with correction for the hemoglobin concentration.

Normal DLCO is usually seen in asthma because, although there is bronchoconstriction, there is no alveolar disease. On the other hand, it may be increased if there is significant bronchospasm or air trapping.

Increased DLCO is also seen in problems that increase effective blood flow to the functional lung, such as heart failure, acute hemorrhage in the lung (i.e., diffuse alveolar hemorrhage), pulmonary infarction, and idiopathic pulmonary hemosiderosis (IPH).

DLCO is not used much. It is sometimes useful for differentiating emphysema from asthma in a younger patient with airflow obstruction.

LUNG VOLUMES AND PULMONARY FUNCTION TESTS

General

In your office, with spirometry, you can determine most of the lung volumes and capacities, expiratory flows, flow-volume loops, and bronchodilator response.

Pulmonary function lab is needed to do:

- total lung capacities
- DLCO
- methacholine or other challenge

In general, < 80% is abnormal. > 120% may also be significant.

Keep in mind while reviewing the following that total lung capacity (TLC) is the function test used to assess interstitial lung disease (i.e., TLC is decreased in restrictive lung disease), and expiratory flow rate (FEV_1/FVC) is used to assess obstructive lung disease.

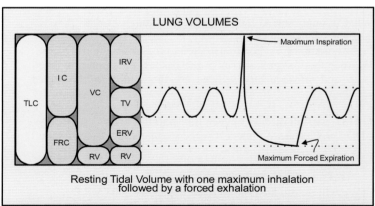

LUNG VOLUMES

Resting Tidal Volume with one maximum inhalation followed by a forced exhalation

Figure 3-2: Lung Volumes

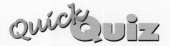

Lung Volumes

Review the Lung Volumes diagram (Figure 3-2, colored highlighting in the following text matches the color of the associated lung volumes colored in this diagram). Note that there are 4 basic functional volumes of which the lung is made:

- residual volume—RV. Unused space
- expiratory reserve volume—ERV—from full non-forced end-expiration to full forced end-expiration
- tidal volume—TV—used in normal unforced ventilation
- inspiratory reserve volume—IRV—from normal unforced end-inspiration to full forced end-inspiration.

A "capacity" is equal to ≥ 2 of these basic volumes and gives an even more functional significance to them. Note that the vital capacity (VC) is composed of the IRV + TV + ERV. The total lung capacity (TLC) is composed of the VC + RV.

In severe COPD, the total lung capacity is normal or increased (even though vital capacity is decreased) due to a greatly increased RV—seen as barrel chest. In restrictive disease, the TLC is decreased due to both a decreased VC and RV.

The tracing in the Lung Volumes diagram shows a forced expiration from maximum inspiration. The next diagram (Figure 3-3) shows a comparison of similar expirations for patients with normal, obstructive, and restrictive airways. This is an easy and important test, but usually you will not see it diagrammed this way.

Although the TLC cannot be determined from spirometry (must know the RV), you can determine the degree of obstruction by comparing the forced volume expired at 1 second (FEV_1) to the forced vital capacity in the ratio FEV_1/FVC (FVC is just the VC during a forced expiration). In a patient with a normal lung, the ratio is about 0.8. It is always less in a COPD patient or an asthma patient having an acute attack, but may be normal or increased in a patient with restrictive disease—even though the VC is small—because this patient has no trouble getting air out. A patient with asthma has reversible disease and, if not having an acute attack, may have a normal FEV_1/FVC.

TLC is determined in the lab by helium dilution, nitrogen washout, or plethysmography. Use plethysmography for patients with airflow obstruction.

Flow-Volume Loops

The diagrams of flow-volume loops shown are a more common way of expressing airflow in the different lung diseases—again, these are derived from the spirometry data, and are calculated and plotted by an attached computer, where the FEV_1/FVC is automatically determined. Note that the y-axis is flow rate.

Because we cannot determine RV from spirometry, we get most of our information by the shape of the loop. The exception is in restrictive disease; the shape is similar to normal,

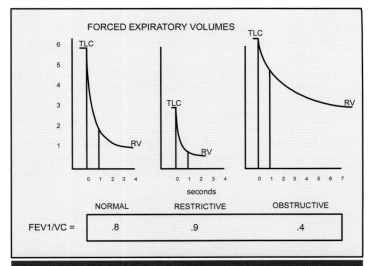

Figure 3-3: Forced Expiratory Volumes and FEV_1/VC

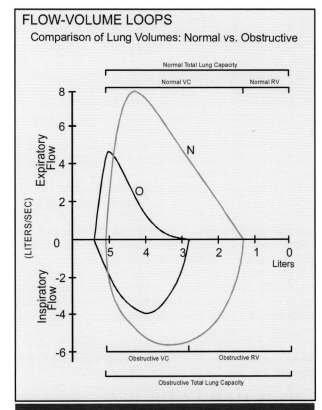

Figure 3-4: Flow-Volume Loop—Obstruction 1

notes

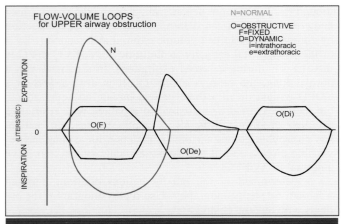

Figure 3-5: Flow-Volume Loops—Obstruction 2

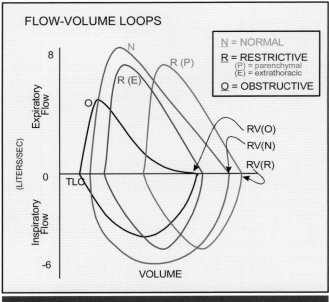

Figure 3-6: Flow-Volume Loops—All

but the vital capacity (= TLC - RV) is much smaller than normal.

Figure 3-4 compares obstructive vs. normal lung flow loops. Figure 3-5 compares the different types of obstructive disease. Figure 3-6 includes restrictive diseases.

When analyzing an obstructive disease of the upper airway (from the pharynx to the origin of the mainstem bronchi), you can derive much information from the shape of the flow-volume loop. See Figure 3-5.

Fixed upper airway obstruction: If the upper airway obstruction is fixed, the graph is flattened on the bottom and the top; i.e., during both inspiration and expiration. Examples of fixed obstruction are conditions due to compressive tumors (e.g., thyroid tumors) and tracheal stenosis (e.g., history of intubation).

Dynamic upper airway obstruction: With dynamic extrathoracic obstruction, such as in tracheomalacia and vocal cord paralysis, the obstruction occurs on inspiration (think of a thin rubber wall instead of the normal trachea in the neck collapsing from the negative pressure of inspiration).

If the tracheomalacia is intrathoracic, the flow is impeded on expiration (due to the increased intrathoracic pressure pressing on the malacic trachea).

The flow rate midway through inspiration is called FIF_{50}, while mid-expiratory flow rate is called FEF_{50}. Notice that $FEF_{50}/FIF_{50} = 1$ in patients with normal function or fixed upper airway obstruction; it is < 1 in intrathoracic dynamic obstruction and > 1 in extrathoracic dynamic obstruction.

Increased expiratory airway resistance causes decreased expiratory flow rate. Again, while normal $FEV_1/FVC = 80\%$, in obstruction it may be only 40%! Additionally, there is a scooping of the tracing in the latter half of expiration. Causes of lower airway obstruction include asthma, COPD, bronchiectasis, and cystic fibrosis.

Bronchodilator response during pulmonary function testing is done for 2 reasons:
1) To determine if the obstruction is responsive to beta-agonists. Before testing, hold beta$_2$-agonists for 8 hours and theophylline 12–24 hours.

2) To test for efficacy of current regimen. In this case, medications are not held. If treated patients have a response to beta$_2$-agonists, it suggests that they are not on an optimum regimen.

Methacholine or other bronchoprovocation-challenge testing is done in people with intermittent asthma-like symptoms, or other symptoms suggestive of airflow obstruction, to determine if they have bronchial hyperreactivity This test is often done in the workup of chronic cough (see Asthma on pg 3-8). Inhaled methacholine (or histamine or cold air) is given to the patient—while looking for a 20% drop in FEV_1. Asthmatics will reach this 80% level at a very low dose of the irritant, whereas a non-asthmatic may never drop that low.

PFTs are not indicated in the routine pre-op exam.

PFTs + ABGs are indicated in the following circumstances:
1) If the surgical procedure is close to the diaphragm (gallbladder, etc.).
2) If the patient has moderate or worse lung disease. In these cases, a $FEV_1 < 1$ liter or an elevated pCO_2 indicates that the patient is at risk for post-op pulmonary complications.
3) Lung cancer or lung resection surgery pre-surgical evaluation. Assuming a worst-case scenario (pneumonectomy), the patient must still have adequate lung function post-op. High risk of post-op morbidity is indicated by a predicted $FEV_1 \leq 0.8$ L after surgery. In a patient with a pre-op $FEV_1 \leq 1.6$ L, you can estimate the post-op FEV_1 by doing split-lung PFTs (hard to do), obtaining a quantitative ventilation, or by quantitative perfusion lung scan. Then multiply the % perfusion (or ventilation) of what will be left after surgery by the FEV_1 to obtain the estimated post-op FEV_1.

notes

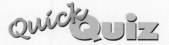

1) Be able to identify flow-volume loop for restrictive and obstructive (dynamic and static) airway diseases.
2) When is methacholine bronchoprovocation testing performed?
3) In restrictive lung disease, what happens always to the TLC?
4) Know the typical PFT results for different lung diseases, and know why these results occur.

Now, let's first look at what PFTs show in the major lung diseases. In subsequent sections, we will focus on the clinical aspects of the major lung diseases.

PFTs for Specific Lung Diseases

I) Emphysema:
- decreased expiratory flow (shortened height of top portion of the flow-volume loop)
- concave expiratory flow-volume loop tracing
- minimal response to beta$_2$-agonist: < 12% improvement *or* < 200 ml improvement in FEV$_1$ or FVC
- increased TLC, reduced VC (hyperinflation with trapped air)
- decreased DLCO (destruction of alveolar-capillary interface—suggests emphysema)

II) Chronic bronchitis:
- decreased expiratory flow (shortened height of top portion of the flow-volume loop)
- concave expiratory flow-volume loop tracing
- minimal response to beta$_2$-agonist: < 12% improvement *or* < 200 ml improvement in FEV$_1$ or FVC
- normal or only slight increase in TLC = normal or slightly reduced VC
- DLCO is normal or slightly reduced (much lower in emphysema)

III) Asthma: may be normal or:
- decreased expiratory flow (shortened height of top portion of the flow-volume loop)
- concave expiratory flow-volume loop tracing
- significant response to beta$_2$-agonist
- normal or increased TLC (due to hyperinflation) = normal or reduced VC
- DLCO is normal or slightly increased (due to air-trapping)

IV) Interstitial lung disease:
- mildly decreased expiratory flow, but slightly increased when compared to normals at the same lung volume—i.e., FEV$_1$/FVC may be normal or supranormal
- straight or slightly convex expiratory flow-volume loop tracing
- proportional decrease in all lung volumes

- DLCO is reduced (due to thickening of the alveolar-capillary interface)

Now some examples. When evaluating a PFT scenario, think in terms of:
- expiratory flow
- lung volumes
- diffusion capacity
- response to bronchodilators

Also consider that anything < 80% of normal is an abnormal finding (FEV$_1$/FVC is already age-adjusted).

Approach to PFT results analysis. We will be using Table 3-1 during this discussion. Remember, we are basically looking for normal, restrictive, or obstructive disease.

Note: Each time you figure out a line, label it.

1) <u>Look for all normals</u>:
   Circle everything ≥ 80%—these values are "normal." If all values are ≥ 80%, the results are normal. Label it "normal." Remember that most smokers are normal.

2) <u>Look for restrictive disease</u>:
   Any TLC < 80% is, by definition, restrictive. Label these results as "restrictive." If TLC is not known, restrictive disease is reflected in a proportional decrease in FEV$_1$ and FVC (i.e., FEV$_1$/FVC = 80% but FVC is < 80%).
   If restrictive, check the DLCO: This will determine if it is extrathoracic or intrathoracic:
   - If the decrease in DLCO is proportional to the decrease in TLC, it means that the restriction is not due to parenchymal disease—rather, it is of extrathoracic origin. Label it "extrathoracic" and think of obesity and kyphosis.
   - If the decrease in DLCO is disproportionately low compared to the decrease in TLC, label it "intrathoracic" and "ILD" (interstitial lung disease).

3) <u>Look for obstructive disease</u>:
   Obstruction is defined by a disproportionately low FEV$_1$. So both FEV$_1$ and FEV$_1$/FVC are low. Label these lines "obstructive."
   If obstructive, check the TLC, DLCO, and reaction to beta$_2$-agonist:
   - "Emphysema" if the TLC is high but the DLCO is low. No reaction to beta$_2$-agonist.
   - "Asthma" if the DLCO is normal, or there typically is a reaction to beta$_2$-agonist.

4) <u>Others are combinations</u> of obstructive and restrictive diseases. Especially seen in patients with combined problems (asthma + obesity) or with certain lung diseases, especially sarcoidosis, eosinophilic granuloma (Histiocytosis X), and lymphangioleiomyomatosis.

Okay, let's apply this to a table of PFT results. In your practice (or on your boards), you may or may not have these same test results. Table 3-1 reviews some PFT results as a percentage of predicted. Remember that, in general and especially for the boards, < 80% of predicted is abnormal.

notes

Table 3-1: PFT Analysis Table

	%FEV1	%FVC	%TLC	%DLCO
1	83	89	92	85
2	58	62	68	64
3	52	80	110	65
4	55	87	100	88
5	57	82	70	68
6	66	72	75	66

1) You should have all these values circled. These are, of course, normal. Remember that normal results are seen in most smokers!

2) Extrathoracic restrictive mechanics (i.e., non-parenchymal). All restrictions are defined by a decrease in the TLC. That there is no other mechanism involved is shown by the maintenance of FEV_1/FVC ratio: the FEV_1 is decreased in proportion to the decrease in FVC, so the $FEV_1/FVC > 80\%$. The extrathoracic involvement is indicated by the proportional decrease in TLC and DLCO. Pure extrathoracic restriction is seen with kyphoscoliosis and obesity. Although kyphoscoliosis occurs in a small percentage of neurofibromatosis patients (Von Recklinghausen disease) and may be due to tuberculosis involving the thoracic vertebrae, it is usually a result of compression fractures of the thoracic vertebral bodies, secondary to long-standing osteoporosis.

Note: If a patient is 1–3 days post-CABG and suffering from orthopnea, check the PFTs, but also check FVC both standing and lying down. If the patient has extrathoracic restrictive mechanics and the difference in FVC is > 20% (decreases with lying down), consider bilateral diaphragmatic paralysis from the cold cardioplegia. (This is for board questions—a chest x-ray could have told you this!) Unilateral phrenic nerve problems can be diagnosed by a "sniff test" with fluoroscopy. Also note that a decrease in FVC (from standing to lying) in the high-normal range (15–20%) is commonly seen with obesity. The DLCO could be disproportionately low (say, 54%) if this post-CABG patient also had some post-op atelectasis.

Question: Besides cold cardioplegia, what are other possible causes of bilateral elevated hemidiaphragm? Answer: Poor inspiration, SLE, bilateral phrenic nerve paralysis (spine injury, tumor, neurological disorder), diaphragmatic weakness from ALS, large-volume ascites, bilateral subpulmonic effusions. These all make sense, so just think about them, but don't memorize them!

3) Pure obstruction with low DLCO and a high TLC. The $FEV_1/FVC < 80\%$. The TLC is high and the DLCO is disproportionately low, indicating a loss of alveolar-capillary units. Most probable etiology is emphysema—from either smoking or α-1 antitrypsin deficiency.

4) Pure obstruction with normal DLCO. Same as #3, except the DLCO is normal, indicating asthma. In both #3 and #4, you may find a low FVC if the obstruction is so severe, the patient does not have enough time to fully expire before getting short of breath.

5) Combined obstruction and extrathoracic restriction. The low FEV_1/FVC indicates obstruction. The low TLC indicates restriction, while the proportionate decrease in DLCO narrows it to an extrathoracic etiology. Possible etiologies: an obese patient with asthma or an osteoporotic kyphotic patient with asthma.

6) Intrathoracic restriction. As in extrathoracic restriction, the FEV_1 and FVC are both low ($FEV_1/FVC > 80\%$). Contrary to extrathoracic restriction, in intrathoracic restriction the DLCO is disproportionately lower than the decrease in TLC. Intrathoracic restriction is seen with many interstitial lung diseases.

OBSTRUCTIVE LUNG DISEASES
ASTHMA

Overview

Asthma is basically a reversible, inflammatory condition of the airways with a multifactorial etiology. The inflammatory response has an acute phase and a late phase. Some asthma is IgE-mediated. Most asthmatics, whatever the etiology, develop a nonspecific airway hyperresponsivity, as shown by exacerbations due to cold, dust, and viral infections. Additionally, these people react to the methacholine challenge done with pulmonary function tests. The reaction to dust is more specifically a reaction to the dust mite.

First, we will discuss regular asthma and then exercise-induced asthma.

Early in an asthmatic attack, bronchospasm is the major factor; but later on, airway inflammation, airway edema, and increased airway secretions with possible mucous plugging may dominate—especially suspect this in status asthmaticus. Asthmatics usually present with some combination of dyspnea, cough, and wheezing but, on the initial presentation, the patient may have complaints only of a chronic cough (remember that patients with GERD may also present with a cough, but cough due to GE reflux disease occurs only when supine). Regarding patients with a fatal asthma attack, the main factor in mortality is the amount of auto-PEEP they experience.

Persistent airway inflammation may lead to remodeling of the airways due to fibrosis, etc., resulting in a persistent nonresponsive asthma as a component of the clinical picture.

Severity of asthma is categorized as mild intermittent, mild persistent, moderate persistent, and severe persistent. Any severity level can have exacerbations—which in turn may be mild, moderate, or severe.

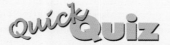
A very interesting aspect of asthma is its relationship to GERD. Presence of GE reflux can exacerbate asthma—especially at night. Asthmatics with GERD are more likely to cough during the asthma attack. About 80% of hard-to-control asthmatics improve with antireflux therapy! Also about 80% of asthmatics have abnormal esophageal acid contact times—and 30% of these patients have no symptoms! Conversely, asthma and its treatment may exacerbate GERD by decreasing LES pressure.

The cause of asthma is often not discovered, especially in adult-onset asthma.

Some specifics: occupational causes—e.g., isocyanates (most common!), cotton dust (byssinosis), toluene diisocyanate, fluorocarbons, grain dust, and wood dust (especially western cedar). But not silica! …and don't forget GERD.

ASA-sensitive asthmatics may also be sensitive to other NSAIDs and tartrazine dyes, but not to sodium or choline salicylates.

Asthma Triad: • ASA sensitivity + • asthma + • nasal polyposis; but patients usually have just 2 of the 3 findings.

Occupational asthma may be IgE-dependent (causes an early or biphasic reaction) or IgE-independent (late reaction). Both smoking and a history of atopy are important sensitizing factors for occupational asthma.

Triggers may be the cause of asthma or something that induces worsening symptoms when the airways are hypersensitive. Triggers can be broadly categorized into 6 areas: allergens, irritants, chemicals, respiratory infections, physical stress, and emotional stress.

Diagnosis of Asthma

Diagnosis: the patient demonstrates at least partially reversible bronchospasm and a history compatible with asthma. Only if these are not demonstrated do you do a challenge test to induce bronchospasm. A common instance when you'd do a challenge test is for a patient with a chronic cough or who has intermittent asthma-like symptoms only by history.

Methacholine challenge (most common test; do not perform in the office!), histamine challenge, and thermal (cold air) chal-

lenge can be used to confirm the diagnosis of asthma. These work on the principle of nonspecific hyperirritability. For the diagnosis of asthma (requires "reversible bronchoconstriction"), the patient must both tighten up with the challenge and loosen up with subsequent bronchodilators. Tests may be coupled (2 or 3 tests at once) with a high index of clinical suspicion for asthma.

Response to a bronchodilator is defined as an increase in FEV_1 or FVC by 12% and 200 cc.

Exercise-induced asthma is diagnosed by a decrease in FEV_1 of $\geq 10\%$ after a thermal challenge—either exercise or hyperventilation.

Treatment of Asthma

Overview

Control or remove the triggers. The most effective treatment for regular asthma is removing the triggering agents. Remove them (e.g., pets) or, if unable, then the patient should minimize contact with them or take extra bronchodilator before exposure.

Because of the strong association of GERD with asthma, many recommend an empiric 3-month trial of a proton pump inhibitor (equivalent to omeprazole, 20 mg bid) if reflux symptoms are present.

Monitor (regularly) peak expiratory flow rate (PEFR) in those with moderate-to-severe asthma.

Pharmacologic treatment when needed. This includes:
1) antiinflammatory meds (corticosteroids, nedocromil)
2) direct bronchodilators (beta$_2$-agonists, anticholinergics, and methylxanthines)
3) mast-cell stabilizer (cromolyn)
4) leukotriene inhibitors/blockers

We'll go over the pharmacologic treatment now.

Pharmacologic Treatment of Asthma

First, we will go over these drugs, then go over the recommended treatment regimens. (See Table 3-2)

1) Antiinflammatory medications.

Corticosteroids:

Inhaled corticosteroids are now the mainstay for chronic maintenance therapy for persistent asthma, and are called "controller medications" for asthma. They are also the initial pharmacologic therapy. Why is this? Asthma is an inflammatory process, and inhaled corticosteroids subdue the inflammation where it occurs—with minimal side effects. Beta$_2$-agonists are merely bronchodilators—i.e., symptomatic treatment.

Twice-per-day inhalations of corticosteroids are as effective as qid; dosage in mild persistent asthmatics often can be reduced to once per day. A spacer greatly reduces the amount of drug deposited in the oropharynx (large particles are trapped in the spacer), thereby decreasing systemic effects from swallowed drug. A spacer also increases the amount of drug reaching the lungs.

notes

Note regarding inhaled corticosteroids: These are safe drugs!
- there is little, if any, effect on the pituitary-adrenal axis
- no increase in fractures
- cataracts are a problem with oral but not inhaled forms
- okay in pregnancy
- may cause easy bruising in elderly patients
- may cause slowing of growth in children, but there is a catch-up period resulting in normal height

Oral corticosteroids are also a great, short-term treatment for an acute exacerbation. They potentiate the effect of beta$_2$-agonists and have an antiinflammatory effect that has been shown to decrease the frequency of returns to the emergency room. Corticosteroid inhalers can be used instead of—or along with—prednisone.

Oral corticosteroids usually provide no benefit for patients with chronic, stable COPD, including no improvement in survival (only oxygen improves survival in this group).

Oral corticosteroids are sufficient for the treatment in the emergency department. Give intravenously only if the patient already has an IV in place. When given IV, the onset of action is 2–6 hours; peak steady state levels occur in 6–8 hours.

Nedocromil (Tilade®) is an inhaled antiinflammatory agent that also has properties similar to cromolyn sodium. Its effectiveness is about the same as cromolyn sodium, and it also takes several weeks to work. Its mechanism of action is prevention of mast cell degranulation. It is not as potent an antiinflammatory medication as steroids.

2) Bronchodilators:

Beta$_2$-agonists act through bronchodilation and do nothing for the underlying swelling or inflammation. Beta$_2$-agonists induce an increase in cAMP, which results in relaxation of the bronchial smooth muscles. Inhalers deliver ~10% of drug to the lungs. Spacer devices slightly increase this amount.

There are several studies indicating a possible problem with regular use of higher-than-normal doses of a long-acting agent (fenoterol). Deaths increased among patients using > 1.4 canisters/month; and the greatest death rate occurred among those with a pattern of increasing usage. It is now thought that this does not necessarily reflect a problem with long-acting beta$_2$-agonists themselves, but rather that their increased use tends to cover up worsening inflammation and the resulting critical need for more corticosteroids or step-up in therapy.

Table 3-2: Treatment of Asthma based on Severity Category

ASTHMA SEVERITY AND TREATMENT (for all patients > 5 yrs old)

SEVERITY	Days with Sx	Nights with Sx	FEV1 or PEF	Tx for Long-term control
1) Mild intermittent	< 3/week	≤ 2/month	≥ 80%	No daily medications
2) Mild persistent	3-6/week	3-4/month	≥ 80%	1) Inhaled low-dose steroid, OR 2) Cromolyn OR 3) Nedocromil 4) Zafirlukast okay if 12 yrs old. Montelukast if > 6 years old. 5) Theophylline is an alternative BUT *not preferred.*
3) Moderate persistent	Daily	≥ 5/month	< 60%, > 80%	1) Inhaled medium-dose steroid OR 2) Inhaled low to med dose steroid plus a long-acting beta$_2$-agonist. Note: If needed, increase to high-dose inhaled steroid PLUS one of the following: a long-acting inhaled beta$_2$-agonist, sustained-release theophylline, or oral beta$_2$-agonist. 3) Anticholinergics, especially if GERD symptoms
4) Severe persistent	Continual	Frequent	≤ 60%	Inhaled high-dose steroids, PLUS Long-acting beta$_2$-agonist PLUS Oral steroids long-term - repeatedly attempt to wean off!

Note1: Review treatment every 1-6 months. If control is maintained for at least 3 months, a stepdown may be possible.

Note2: All acute exacerbations are treated with 2-4 puffs of a short-acting inhaled beta$_2$-agonist every 20 minutes x 3 max. A short course of oral steroids may be needed.

Note3: This table adapted from "Stepwise Approach to Managing Asthma for Adults and Children More than 5 Years of Age." NIH publication No. 99-4055A.

notes

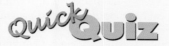

Inhaled, short-acting beta$_2$-agonists are the first choice for treatment of an acute exacerbation of asthma, even if the patient routinely uses them at home. Treatment for acute exacerbations is termed "rescue treatment."

Use inhaled, long-acting beta$_2$-agonists routinely for moderate-to-severe asthma—but not for mild asthma and not for acute treatment. Warn the patient to consult you before increasing the dose of this drug (see above).

Long-acting beta-agonists are reported to have mild antiinflammatory activity, and may also be helpful in preventing exercise-induced asthma (EIA).

Anticholinergics: Atropine and ipratropium bromide (Atrovent®). These are more effective than beta$_2$-agonists only in patients with COPD. Anticholinergics cause a decrease in cGMP that relaxes contractions of bronchial smooth muscle. They are usually given along with beta$_2$-agonists for acute exacerbations of COPD. There are suggestions that they may be effective as an adjunctive drug in asthma precipitated by sulfur dioxide air pollution, cold air, stress, and cigarette smoke. Not very useful in most asthmatics. Ipratropium is helpful in patients with GERD + Asthma because bronchospasm is mediated by vagal fibers.

Theophylline, a methylxanthine, is less effective than beta$_2$-agonists. Mechanism of action is uncertain but is probably inhibition of phosphodiesterase and its isozymes. Theophylline appears to down-regulate autoimmune and inflammatory functions. Unfortunately, the dose-response curve for theophylline is log-linear and, therefore, has a narrow therapeutic index and increased risk for toxicity.

In an acute asthma attack, if large doses of beta$_2$-agonists are being given, adding theophylline does not help. It is not very useful in typical asthmatics.

Theophylline does have a use in young, chronic, asthmatic children or adults who do not tolerate or comply with the inhaled meds and who require maintenance treatment.

In maintenance COPD usage, it has an additive effect with beta$_2$-agonists. It may improve diaphragmatic muscle strength. See the General Internal Medicine section for treatment of theophylline overdose.

Theophylline is no longer a first-line drug for asthma or COPD management—now more like 3rd or 4th line.

3) Cromolyn sodium is not a bronchodilator and has no anticholinergic activity. It is a mast cell stabilizer and inhibits induced degranulation of mast cells. It has mild antiinflammatory activity by modifying release of inflammatory mediators. It is most effective in young, atopic asthmatics. No toxicity. It is not effective during acute bronchospasm. Indeed, it takes several weeks to establish effectiveness.

Remember nedocromil, (Tilade®) discussed in "1" above, is a mild, inhaled antiinflammatory agent that also has properties similar to cromolyn sodium.

4) Antileukotriene drugs are a new class of anti-asthma drug. Arachidonic acid is released from stimulated mast cells, basophils, and eosinophils. It is then partially metabolized into leukotrienes, which are potent:
- smooth muscle contractors
- promoters of mucous production
- causes of airway edema
- vasoconstrictors
- stimulators of more arachidonic acid release

The antileukotriene drugs are ~1/2 as potent as beta$_2$-agonists. Recommended for mild persistent asthma and for asthmatics with "allergies." Generally, not first-line therapy. There are 2 types: receptor antagonists (zafirlukast, montelukast), and synthesis inhibitors (zileuton). You must monitor liver function with zileuton.

Oxygen during an exacerbation of asthma: A P_aO_2 of at least 60 mm Hg or O_2 sat of 90% is the goal.

Management of Asthma

Notes on the Guidelines

The National Asthma Education and Prevention Program (NAEPP) came out with:
Guidelines for the Diagnosis and Management of Asthma. (http://www.nhlbi.nih.gov/guidelines/asthma/index.htm)
Severity of asthma is broken down into 4 levels, with treatment options for each level listed (see Table 3-2). [Know this section!]

Note several points these guidelines make:
1) Asthma is an inflammatory condition, and primary treatment is with inhaled steroids.
2) Give chronic oral steroids only for severe asthma and, even then, repeat attempts to wean off.
3) Use long-term beta$_2$-agonists only for moderate-to-severe asthma.
4) Treat acute exacerbations at any level the same: inhaled short-acting beta$_2$-agonist. Add a short course of oral steroids if there is no improvement, or if the patient has recently been on them (flare-up may be a rebound effect).

notes

Chronic, severe asthma often requires continuous oral prednisone. Steroid-sparing drugs are often tried, and methotrexate may be effective (trials show varying results). Cyclosporine is being investigated. Troleandomycin (TAO), an erythromycin analog, appears to work well at a dose of 250 mg/day.

When an exacerbation occurs, treatment can be "stepped up" one or two levels (per Table 3-2), then slowly "stepped down" until symptoms recur, and then stepped up one level. When treatment is initially started, it is usually started one or two levels above the presumed severity level and then gradually stepped down in the same way.

Note that the older approach of starting low and "stepping up" until symptoms are gone is still valid, just less preferred by the NAEPP expert panel, because the ongoing inflammation is more quickly suppressed with the step-down method.

Management of Exercise-Induced Asthma

Treat exercise-induced asthma with inhaled beta$_2$-agonists 5–60 minutes before exertion. A warm-up period prior to exercise is also helpful. Treat active bronchospasm with warm, moist air and inhaled short-acting beta$_2$-agonists.

Intubation and the Asthma Patient

[Know this topic]

If intubation is required (patient is getting progressively hypercapnic), first sedate and then paralyze. Avoid morphine because it may cause histamine release.

Once intubated, do not bag too quickly! These patients require a prolonged expiration period, and ventilating at too high a rate causes progressive air trapping ("stacking," "auto-PEEP"), which causes decreased venous return or barotrauma (e.g., tension pneumothorax). Decreased venous return → decreased filling pressure → decreased cardiac output, which subsequently → hypotension and poor perfusion of vital organs.

A very important method used when ventilating an asthmatic patient is permissive hypercapnia—a technique of controlled hypoventilation. We no longer try to get the pCO$_2$ down to 40 to resolve the acute respiratory acidosis—this effort in just-intubated asthmatics has had bad outcomes (auto-PEEP)! Initially, focus on maintaining an O$_2$ sat of 90% and don't worry about the pCO$_2$ so much—a reasonable level is 60–70 (even 80) with a serum pH of 7.20–7.25. Besides maintaining an adequate O$_2$ sat, you must ensure that the patient is getting all the air out! Listen with your stethoscope, and check that the ventilator is not kicking in while the patient is still exhaling, or check the waveform analyser on the graphic package of the ventilator.

Ventilator settings: When putting an asthmatic on a ventilator, use a low rate, small tidal volume, and high flows. Each of these addresses the need for a prolonged expiratory phase. High flow on the inspiration allows for less time devoted to inspiration and more to expiration.

COPD

Overview

COPD is usually a mixture of I) emphysema and II) chronic bronchitis, often with predominance of one or the other. III) Peripheral airway disease is another process previously thought to be a distinct entity—now thought to be early emphysema or early chronic bronchitis. There is no abnormal fibrosis in COPD—which distinguishes it from interstitial lung disease. COPD is usually treated with bronchodilators and anticholinergics.

I) Emphysema is the enlargement of the airspace distal to the terminal bronchioles, with destruction of the alveolar septa.
  Centroacinar: Only the area near the terminal bronchiole is affected. This type is usually seen in smokers.
  Panacinar: The entire acinus is affected. Classically seen with α-1 antitrypsin deficiency.
This makes sense because more smoke gets to the proximal portion of the acinus. Bullae appear in the apices of emphysematous smokers and in the bases of people with α-1 antitrypsin deficiency! filling pressure output subsequently hypotension poor perfusion organs
Although most COPD is the result of smoking, < 15% of patients who smoke actually develop emphysema!
Lung mechanics in emphysema: Decreased elastic recoil means increased compliance (and increased TLC). Although there is an increase in TLC, there is an even greater increase in residual volume from air trapping, so the VC (or FVC) is decreased! This air trapping leads to the process of dynamic hyperinflation, and can result in a large amount of auto-PEEP (intrinsic PEEP).
Patients with COPD with emphysema predominance classically are the "pink puffers" because of their reddish complexion and "puffing" hyperventilation.
Auto-PEEP and dynamic hyperinflation occur when the time constant of the lung is violated—as seen in high airway resistance and/or high compliance: Time Constant = R_{airway} x C_L.

II) Chronic bronchitis has a clinical definition, as opposed to the histological definition given for emphysema. It is de-

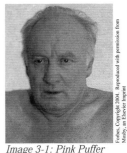

Image 3-1: Pink Puffer

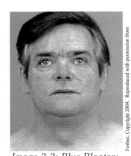

Image 3-2: Blue Bloater; CO$_2$ retainer

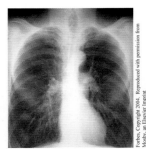

Image 3-3: Cor pulmonale in COPD patient

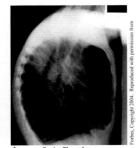

Image 3-4: Emphysema

notes

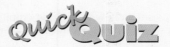

fined as excess bronchial mucous secretion for at least 3 consecutive months for at least 2 years. It occurs in 20% of adult males! One etiology is prolonged irritation by cigarette smoke. Patients may have a bronchospastic component responsive to bronchodilators.

III) Peripheral airway disease results from increased tortuosity, inflammation, and fibrosis. Rather than another entity, it is now thought to be early emphysema/bronchitis. It is often what people are diagnosed with when they don't quite meet the criteria for either emphysema or chronic bronchitis. It is a good disease entity to use to scare smokers into stopping before they develop anything worse.

Of the above 3 components of COPD, the amount of emphysema best correlates with the decrease in airflow seen in COPD patients. The best prognostic indicator in COPD is FEV_1.

In both smokers and nonsmokers, the average decrease in FEV_1 is about 15–30 ml/yr; this is due to normal aging effects. It is only in the minority of smokers that COPD develops. In these susceptible smokers, the lung damage is due to an imbalance in the proteolytic (elastase from neutrophils) and anti-proteolytic (α-1 antitrypsin) activity. These individuals may lose 60–120 ml/yr of lung function.

Again:
- Typical emphysema: centroacinar emphysema; apical bullae; smoking.
- α-1 antitrypsin deficiency: panacinar emphysema; bullae in the bases; smoking greatly accelerates the disease process.

Treatment of COPD:

Acute exacerbations of COPD. The ACP-ASIM and the ACCP co-developed an evidence-based position paper on management of acute exacerbations of COPD (Ann Intern Med. 2001;134:595-599). The gist of the recommendations follows

For all COPD patients presenting to the hospital with an exacerbation:
1) Do a chest x-ray, because up to 23% show new infiltrates that change the chosen therapy.
2) Do not use spirometry to diagnose or assess the severity of an exacerbation.
3) Because inhaled anticholinergic drugs (e.g., ipratropium—Atrovent®) are equally effective and more benign that inhaled beta$_2$-agonists, start treatment with an inhaled anticholinergic drug and move to an inhaled beta$_2$-agonist only after maximum dose of the anticholinergic drug is achieved.

For moderate-to-severe exacerbation:
If the patient has moderate-to-severe exacerbation, consider these therapies, which have shown benefit:
1) Systemic corticosteroids for up to 2 weeks (first IV then oral);
2) NPPV (Noninvasive positive-pressure ventilation); and
3) Oxygen with close observation. (Note that patients with initial abnormal blood gases are at risk for hypercarbia, and subsequent respiratory failure, with supplemental O_2 administration.)

For severe exacerbation:
Antibiotics are recommended, but the position paper is unclear on whether they should be broad- or narrow-spectrum. Most of the studies that showed benefit were done with narrow-spectrum antibiotics, whereas this was before the emergence of multidrug resistant organisms. The Sanford Guide® recommends broader-spectrum treatment: Augmentin®, azithromycin, and extended-spectrum quinolones.

An exercise regimen results in a small but significant improvement in the strength and endurance of respiratory muscle. It does not prolong life.

Oxygen therapy for COPD patients:
The focus of O_2 therapy for COPD patients (or any patient, for that matter) in respiratory distress is to give them enough O_2 to achieve 90% O_2 saturation—or as close as possible (note: O_2sat = oxygen saturation of hemoglobin = S_aO_2 [S_pO_2 if measured with a pulse oximeter]). This is a required endpoint in initial management! Not treating hypoxia causes further end-organ damage, worsening pulmonary vasoconstriction, and a downward spiral to death.

Criteria for starting continuous O_2:
- resting $P_aO_2 < 55$, or
- O_2sat (S_aO_2) $\leq 88\%$, or
- $P_aO_2 < 59$ mm Hg (O_2sat $\geq 89\%$) with evidence of cor pulmonale or erythrocytosis (hematocrit > 55%).

Continuous O_2 use, if needed per the above criteria, increases life span. It is the only treatment modality that decreases morbidity and mortality in severe COPD.

Keep these patients on supplemental O_2 24 hr/d (if not possible, at least 12 hr/d). [Know!]

Intermittent O_2 use: Some patients have similar findings of hypoxia/desat during low-level exercise or sleep. Give these patients supplemental O_2 during these activities. Long-term studies have not been done on this group.

Transtracheal catheters are inconspicuous and, by administering oxygen directly into the trachea, use a lower flow rate. Consider these in patients on chronic O_2. Acceptance by the patient may be an issue.

Associated pulmonary hypertension may develop with as little as 6 hours per day of hypoxia—suspect this entity in:
1) an elderly COPD patient who presents with progressive dyspnea on exertion for several years
2) a patient with a chronic, severe sleep apnea!

Re-evaluate patients placed on oxygen 2 months after they are on a stable regimen of drug therapy—it can be discontinued in up to 40%!

Lung volume-reduction surgery for emphysema was previously done frequently. The idea is that by removing ruined areas of the lung, you decrease the degree of hyperventilation and, thereby, improve chest wall and diaphragm dynamics and mechanical function. Because the procedure was routinely reimbursed, too many were done and outcomes were variable. Trials are underway to determine the best group for this procedure. Later follow-up studies are now available and reveal loss of initial benefit with return of past lung function abnormalities.

CMS (Center for Medicaid and Medicare Services) now pays for LVR surgery performed by an approved center (part of NETT trial) in patients symptomatic despite bronchodilator and pulmonary rehabilitation. Additionally, the most severe group is excluded from approval due to high mortality.

α-1 ANTITRYPSIN DEFICIENCY

More on α-1 antitrypsin deficiency. The alleles responsible for α-1 antitrypsin deficiency occur on a locus called Pi. The most common allele is Pi M. The M means it moves moderately fast on an electrophoretic strip. There are variants of Pi M—some move faster (Pi F) and some slower (Pi Z). Only patients homozygous for the slower allele (Pi^{ZZ}) get severely decreased levels of α-1 antitrypsin. Normal level is 212 +/- 32 mg/dl. Heterozygotes (Pi^{MZ}) have > 80 mg/dl. Homozygotes (Pi^{ZZ}) have ~ 10–20 mg/dl.

Heterozygotes (defined by α-1 antitrypsin level > 80 mg/dl) have no increase in pulmonary disease unless they smoke. Know that ~ 15% of persons with the homozygote Pi^{ZZ} phenotype also get progressive liver fibrosis and cirrhosis—especially common in children. With this type of cirrhosis, as with cirrhosis of any cause, there is an increased incidence of hepatoma.

Suspect homozygous α-1 antitrypsin deficiency in nonsmokers with early onset COPD—typically with the emphysematous bullae in the bases.

Treatment of α-1 antitrypsin deficiency. You can give α-1 antiprotease (pooled human AAT) by weekly IV infusions. It is indicated only for those with an α-1 antitrypsin level < 80 and who exhibit mild-to-moderate obstructive pulmonary mechanics. They should be having pulmonary symptoms before starting treat-

ment because, amazingly, some nonsmoking Pi^{ZZ} genotypes never get the COPD (100% of smokers with Pi^{ZZ} get emphysema at an early age)! Even though IV infusion of α-1 antitrypsin increases blood levels, as yet there is no data showing that it reverses or even stabilizes the lung disease process—in those with moderate obstruction, this treatment does slow the rate of FEV_1 decline and decreases mortality. When the emphysema is severe, the only treatment is lung transplantation.

BRONCHIECTASIS

Bronchiectasis is persistent, pathologic dilatation of the bronchi due to breakdown of the bronchial walls. Suspect it if the patient has a long history of cough with a large amount of purulent, foul-smelling sputum +/- blood. It is almost always caused by infection—usually an acute or recurrent, necrotizing, Gram-negative infection, but occasionally by a chronic, smoldering infection. You frequently see it in old TB areas of involvement.

Bronchiectasis is seen with:
- Cystic fibrosis—most common associated disease state (discussion below).
- Hypogammaglobulinemia—consider this entity with recurrent sinopulmonary infections and chronic cough with purulent sputum. Check IgA, IgM, and IgG (including the IgG subtypes).
- ABPA (acute bronchopulmonary aspergillosis)—associated with bronchiectasis of the upper/central lung fields (see pg 3-20, under Eosinophilic ILDs). ABPA occurs in patients with asthma and some patients with CF.
- Immotile cilia syndromes—e.g., Kartagener, ciliary dysmotility.

You confirm diagnosis of bronchiectasis only by seeing the typical morphologic changes with either a CT scan or bronchogram. A high-resolution CT (HRCT) with 1–2 mm cuts or a helical CT is the method of choice. During the workup, check for low gamma globulin and for high sweat chloride. Staph aureus and Pseudomonas are likely in patients with bronchiectasis due to CF.

Patients with bronchiectasis do benefit from bronchodilators and physiotherapy. Chronic prophylaxis for bronchiectasis does not prevent acute infection or deterioration of pulmonary function.

CYSTIC FIBROSIS

Cystic fibrosis (CF) has a median survival of over 35 years in the U.S. There is an abnormal transfer of Na^+ and Cl^-. Patients produce thick mucous, which is difficult to clear. CF causes sinusitis, bronchiectasis (above), pancreatic insufficiency with occasional portal hypertension, and 2° clubbing. In infants, it causes meconium ileus (10%) and intussuscep-

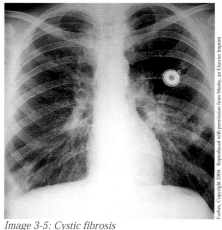

Image 3-5: Cystic fibrosis

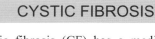

notes

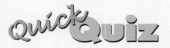

tion. Nasal polyposis, sinusitis, and recurrent pneumonias are common. Most men are infertile (aspermia) and women have difficulty conceiving. In any exam question, if a male patient has fathered a child, he does not have CF. Associated with staphylococcal and pseudomonal infections.

Diagnose CF by demonstrating elevated concentration of chloride and/or sodium in sweat.

You manage CF with bronchodilators, DNase, pancreatic enzymes, mucolytics, physiotherapy, and antibiotics, including inhaled tobramycin for pseudomonal infection. Aerosolized α-1 antitrypsin and amiloride are being evaluated. Bilateral lung transplantation is a treatment option with a 50% 3-year survival.

INTERSTITIAL LUNG DISEASE

OVERVIEW

Interstitial lung diseases (ILD) are a diverse (> 100!) group of disorders that affect the supporting tissue of the lung, especially structural portions of the alveolar walls. The name is partly a misnomer, because there is often bronchial and alveolar involvement. Some call it diffuse parenchymal lung disease (DPLD)—which is more correct. We will call it ILD in this discussion.

The interstitium is usually just a potential space between the capillaries and the alveoli. With ILDs, there is early alveolar disease with later collagen deposition in the interstitium (scarring), which often secondarily changes the architecture of the alveoli and airways.

ILDs also have common factors in their clinical presentation: dyspnea, diffuse disease on x-ray, restrictive PFTs, and an elevated A-a gradient.

ILDs can be most easily grouped into those of known cause and those that are idiopathic. Those of known causes are usually due to dust (organic or inorganic) from occupational or environmental exposures. We will now discuss the following general groupings of these ILDs:

I)   Occupational and environmental causes of ILD
II) Idiopathic interstitial pneumonias (IIP)
III) Other causes of ILD

I) ILDs: OCCUPATIONAL AND ENVIRONMENTAL

Overview

There are 3 categories of occupational/environmental ILDs:
1) Hypersensitivity pneumonitis
2) Organic dust induced: byssinosis
3) Inorganic dust induced: asbestosis, silicosis, coal workers pneumoconiosis, and berylliosis
We will now discuss each of these.

Hypersensitivity Pneumonitis

Hypersensitivity pneumonitis is an immune-mediated granulomatous reaction to organic antigens. As such, not many people get it—just those susceptible to it. Poorly formed granulomas are typical (the granulomas in sarcoidosis are much denser). It has a wide range of causes and, especially on the history taking, the occupation of the patient often leads to the cause. The various causes include:
• moldy hay (thermophilic actinomycetes), aka "farmer's lung"
• pet birds, aka "bird-fancier's lung"
• grain dust (workers in a grain elevator)
• isocyanates
• air conditioning systems

It has acute, subacute, and chronic forms with a typically insidious onset. Consider hypersensitivity pneumonitis in patients with "recurrent or persistent pneumonias."

Diagnose by history. Chest x-ray may reveal recurrent infiltrates, but these are fleeting. Serum precipitins are nonspecific for hypersensitivity pneumonitis because these indicate only exposure, and most people exposed to these antigens have no immune reaction.

Differential diagnoses include other causes of "recurrent or persistent pneumonias:" eosinophilic pneumonia and cryptogenic organizing pneumonia (COP = idiopathic BOOP).

Best treatment is to remove the patient from the offending antigen. Corticosteroids are beneficial only in acute disease.

Organic Dusts that Cause ILD: Byssinosis

Byssinosis is caused by inhalation of cotton, flax, or hemp dust. Not immune-related, no sensitization needed. Early stage has occasional chest tightness; late stage has regular chest tightness toward the end of the first day of the workweek ("Monday chest tightness"). The frequency of symptoms slowly increases to include more days.

Inorganic Dusts that Cause ILD

Overview

These ILDs are: asbestosis, silicosis, coal workers' pneumoconiosis, and berylliosis.

Asbestos

Asbestos exposure (not asbestosis) causes bilateral, **mid-**thoracic pleural thickening/plaque/calcification formation. The pleural thickening usually involves the **mid**-thorax (posterolateral) and spares both the costophrenic angles and the apices. On the chest x-ray, asbestos exposure looks like (and is often discussed as) diaphragmatic calcification with sparing of the costophrenic angle. Remember that pleural plaques and pleural thickening are completely benign; they are not manifestations of asbestosis.

The most common manifestation of asbestos exposure in the first 10 years is benign asbestos pleural effusions (BAPE). These vary from serous to bloody and tend to occur early in the exposure history (within 5 years). 1/3 have eosinophilia of the pleural fluid.

Malignant mesotheliomas are associated (80%) with asbestos exposure (again, merely exposure—not necessarily asbestosis!) It is a tumor arising from the mesothelial cell of the pleura—the area affected by asbestos exposure. Latency period can be > 40 years. It is not associated with smoking. It is usually a rapidly fatal disease.

Asbestosis is the pulmonary disease—the parenchymal fibrosis and resultant impairment caused by prolonged exposure to asbestos. The pulmonary parenchymal fibrosis develops mostly in the bases. Asbestosis generally occurs with > 10 years of moderate exposure, although the latency period is > 30 years! Smoking has a synergistic effect with asbestosis in the development of lung cancer. The associated lung cancers are squamous and adeno—but not small- or large-cell! No specific treatment.

Silica

Silicosis is the most prevalent occupational disease in the world. It requires years of exposure to crystalline silica to develop—as in mining, glassmaking, ceramics, sandblasting, foundries, and brick yards—with a latency of 20–30 years. Simple nodular silicosis (i.e., small nodules) is "fibro-calcific" and usually involves the upper lung, so the differential diagnosis includes TB, coal workers pneumoconiosis, and berylliosis. Silicosis is associated with these silicotic nodules, involvement of the hilar lymph nodes ("hilar eggshell calcification"), and increased susceptibility to TB. You should do yearly PPDs in these patients.

Silica ingested by alveolar macrophages renders them ineffective—so a +PPD in these patients should receive prophylaxis no matter what the patient's age or duration of +PPD.

No specific treatment for silicosis but, if symptoms are rapidly worsening, think TB.

Note: Asbestosis involves the lower lung. There is probably a slight association of silicosis with adenocarcinoma of the lung (being debated!). Silicosis does not cause asthma.

Complicated, nodular silicosis (i.e., big nodules; also called progressive, massive fibrosis) has nodules > 1 cm, which tend to coalesce. Overwhelming exposure leads to silico-proteinosis in ~ 5 years—which results in alveolar filling with eosinophilic material similar to that found in pulmonary alveolar proteinosis (pg 3-21). These patients present with symptoms easily mistaken as pulmonary edema.

Coal

Coal workers' pneumoconiosis (CWP) also has simple and progressive forms. The chest x-ray shows upper lung field nodules (similar to silicosis and berylliosis). Progression of simple CWP correlates with the amount of coal dust deposited in the lungs, whereas complicated CWP does not. Complicated CWP is a progressive massive fibrosis defined by nodules > 2 cm (no hilar involvement). With large depositions of coal dust, patients have melanoptysis. As expected, cigarette smoking accelerates the deterioration of pulmonary function. No association with TB. No specific treatment.

Caplan syndrome is seropositive rheumatoid arthritis associated with massive CWP. This syndrome is heralded by the development of peripheral lung nodules (in addition to the upper-lung field nodules seen in CWP).

Beryllium

Berylliosis is caused by a cell-mediated immune response that can occur from ≥ 2-year exposure to even slight amounts of beryllium. Especially suspect in persons working in high-tech electronics, alloys, ceramics, the Manhattan Project nuclear program, and pre-1950 fluorescent light manufacturing.

It usually causes a chronic interstitial pneumonitis, which tends to affect the upper lobes (like silicosis, TB, and CWP). Pa-

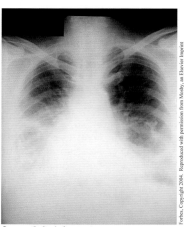

Image 3-6: Asbestosis

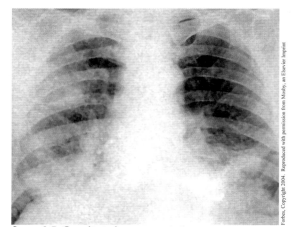

Image 3-7: Complicated pneumoconiosis

notes

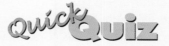

tients often have hilar lymphadenopathy that looks identical on chest x-ray to that caused by sarcoidosis. If the signs and symptoms are suggestive, diagnose berylliosis by the beryllium lymphocyte transformation test.

This one can be treated! Corticosteroids are very effective.

II) ILDs: IDIOPATHIC INTERSTITIAL PNEUMONIAS (IIPs)

Overview

We will now discuss the second category of ILDs—idiopathic interstitial pneumonias (IIPs). Here is a listing in order of occurrence:
- idiopathic pulmonary fibrosis (IPF)
- nonspecific interstitial pneumonia (NSIP)
- cryptogenic organizing pneumonia (COP, idiopathic BOOP)
- acute interstitial pneumonia (AIP)
- respiratory bronchiolitis-associated ILD (RB-ILD)
- desquamative interstitial pneumonia (DIP)
- lymphocytic interstitial pneumonia (LIP)

Each of these entities has specific histopathologic findings, and IPF also has typical clinical and radiologic findings. We will discuss the two most prominent IIPs.

Idiopathic Pulmonary Fibrosis (IPF)

As its name implies, the etiology of idiopathic pulmonary fibrosis (IPF) is uncertain, although it is thought to be autoimmune. IPF is a diagnosis of exclusion. It accounts for up to 50% of ILDs. There are no extrapulmonary manifestations of this disease. M = F, average age = 55 yrs, but it occurs in all age groups; smoking exacerbates the disease. ~ 10% of patients may have low titers of ANA or RF.

IPF, by definition, has the specific histopathologic findings of usual interstitial pneumonia (UIP).

IPF ranges from an early inflammatory stage, amenable to treatment, to an untreatable late fibrotic stage with severe restrictive disease, pulmonary hypertension, and cor pulmonale.

Early IPF is characterized by "leakiness" of the capillaries and alveolar wall (from damage to the capillary endothelial cells and the adjacent Type I squamous alveolar cells) → which causes interstitial and alveolar edema → which ultimately causes intraalveolar hyaline membranes.

The fluid in the alveoli and in the interstitial edema has increased numbers of alveolar macrophages. These release cytokines and pro-inflammatory mediators (tumor necrosis factor (TNF), interleukin 8, and leukotriene B_4)—some of which attract neutrophils. High-resolution CT (HRCT) in early IPF shows a "ground glass" appearance of the alveoli. This is reflected in bronchoalveolar lavage (BAL) results of increased macrophages, neutrophils (PMNs = 20%), and eosinophils (2–4%).

Late IPF leads to increasing alveolar-capillary permeability, desquamation of the alveolar wall, and fibrosis.

Presentation: Suspect IPF in patients presenting with dyspnea, cough, and a diffuse infiltrative process on chest x-ray. Other than clubbing (which is common), the patient has no extrapulmonary signs or symptoms, and history relates no associations with infection, drugs, or chemicals. The patient has a history of progressive exercise intolerance, and auscultation generally reveals coarse, dry crackles at the lung bases. The chest x-ray changes correlate poorly with disease activity but generally show diffuse reticular or reticulonodular disease. Like many ILDs, PFTs show a "restrictive-intrathoracic" disease (low TLC, nl FEV_1/FVC, low DLCO).

Diagnostic workup includes: Chest x-ray, HRCT, PFTs, ABG, and a histologic tissue diagnosis. About 50% of patients with the typical clinical and HRCT findings are consistent with UIP.

You can confirm diagnosis of IPF in ~ 25% of patients by transbronchial biopsy revealing UIP. If transbronchial biopsy is not sufficient, order a thorascopic-guided lung biopsy or open lung biopsy, especially when there is any suggestion that there may be an infection involved, or in younger patients.

Avoid lung biopsy if the patient has negative environmental and drug history, is > 70 years old, has clubbing, coarse crackles, and honeycombed lungs.

Note: Infection and cancer are the 2 most serious mimicking diseases to rule out since immunosuppressives are not helpful in either, and may be extremely harmful.

A bronchoscopy with transbronchial biopsy and lavage can rule out sarcoidosis and lymphangitic cancer fairly well. With early IPF, the BAL fluid has the nonspecific finding of a large number of WBCs—predominance of neutrophils is a bad sign, while lymphocyte predominance is more favorable.

Treatment: This disease progresses to death. With treatment, corticosteroids +/- cyclophosphamide or azathioprine, ~ 20–30% of patients show some improvement. These are usually the patients with early IPF, in which there is a suppressible inflammatory component. Short-term response to corticosteroids is the best prognostic indicator available. The best test for determining improvement is measurement of lung function—lung volumes, DLCO, and ABGs (A-a gradient), in-

notes

cluding the A-a gradient response to exercise. Cor pulmonale is treated symptomatically, but new treatments under investigation include γ-interferon, bosentan, and pirfenidone. Single-lung transplantation is an option for some late-IPF patients.

Give IPF patients pneumococcal and influenza vaccines.

Cryptogenic Organizing Pneumonia

Cryptogenic organizing pneumonia (COP = idiopathic bronchiolitis obliterans organizing pneumonia = idiopathic BOOP) is a very specific entity with an unknown cause. COP is a bronchiolitis (inflammation of the small airways) and a chronic alveolitis (the organizing pneumonia). The bronchiolitis causes a proliferation of granulation tissue within the small airways and alveolar ducts. In adults, it is associated with penicillamine use and, independently, with rheumatoid arthritis (i.e., RA not treated with penicillamine).

Common presentation of COP is an insidious onset (weeks to 1–2 months) of cough, fever, dyspnea, malaise, and myalgias. Often, patients have had multiple courses of antibiotics without effect. Rales are common. Chest x-ray shows some interstitial disease, bronchial thickening, and patchy bilateral alveolar infiltrate.

You must differentiate COP from IPF, because COP has a good prognosis and responds to steroids. To differentiate COP from IPF: IPF is even more insidious in onset (> 6 months), and the patients do not have fever (see Table 3-3). Open lung biopsy is the definitive means of diagnosing COP.

Corticosteroids are the treatment of choice. COP does not respond to antibiotics. Slowly taper corticosteroids over ~ 6 months.

Table 3-3: Comparison of COP and IPF

Cryptogenic Organizing Pneumonia vs. Idiopathic Pulmonary Fibrosis		
	COP	IPF
Signs	Acutely ill appearing; fever	NOT acutely ill appearing; NO fever
Onset of sx	Days to weeks	Very SLOW - at least 6 months
Chest x-ray	Patchy infiltrates	DIFFUSE infiltrates

III) OTHER CAUSES OF ILD

Overview

Other causes of ILD and diffuse lung disease are:
- collagen-vascular diseases
- sarcoidosis
- eosinophilic granuloma
- lymphangioleiomyomatosis
- vasculitides causing ILD: Wegener's, lymphomatoid, Churg-Strauss, bronchocentric, and PAN
- eosinophilic ILDs: eosinophilic pneumonia, ABPA
- alveolar proteinosis
- idiopathic pulmonary hemosiderosis
- Goodpasture syndrome

Collagen Vascular Diseases that Cause ILD

ILD in patients with collagen vascular diseases. Brief notes here highlight the important topics:

> 1/3 of patients with rheumatoid arthritis (RA) get ILD! The most common lung problem in RA is pleurisy (with or without pleural effusion). Pleural effusions are exudative with a very low glucose level (see pleural effusions on pg 3-29). Occasionally, these patients have necrobiotic nodules—usually in the upper lung zones. ILD can also be due to a complication of gold and methotrexate treatment in the RA patients, while COP (discussed above) may rarely result from penicillamine treatment.

SLE also causes painful pleuritis +/- effusion, but additionally causes diffuse atelectasis and sometimes diaphragmatic weakness (and therefore, orthopneic dyspnea that is out of proportion to the chest x-ray findings; although the chest x-ray may show elevated diaphragms). It also occasionally causes hemoptysis similar to that in idiopathic pulmonary hemosiderosis. SLE affects both lung and pleura more frequently than any other CT disease (60%), while scleroderma affects the lung alone more than any (100%! But no pleural changes). So not much in the way of differences between ILD with SLE!

Scleroderma has 3 lung effects:
1) interstitial fibrosis, as just mentioned,
2) intimal proliferation, and
3) potential for lung injury from recurrent aspiration 2° achalasia.

It is this intimal proliferation in the pulmonary artery that causes pulmonary hypertension out of proportion to the pulmonary disease. So, it is not the ILD, but the intimal proliferation that cause the real pulmonary problem in scleroderma patients. Patients with scleroderma are more susceptible to pneumonia. Both RA and scleroderma are associated with exposure to silica, and both have an increased incidence of bronchogenic carcinoma!

Sjögren's causes desiccation of the airways and is also associated with lymphocytic interstitial pneumonia (LIP).

Sarcoidosis

Sarcoidosis: "noncaseating granuloma" is a multisystem disease. Chest x-ray findings are variable. Usually, there is bilateral hilar and/or mediastinal adenopathy +/- reticulonodular or alveolar infiltrates. PFTs may either be normal or show restrictive +/- obstructive mechanics. The radiographic staging of sarcoidosis (see Table 3-4) illustrates the interesting point that hilar adenopathy disappears as the disease progresses. Serum angiotensin-converting enzyme level (SACE) is nonspecific and considered of no use in diagnosis, but it may be useful for monitoring progression of disease (controversial). If it was previously elevated when the disease was active, and low when inactive, SACE levels may be useful in determining if the disease is once again active. Hyper-

notes

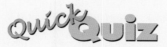

calcemia, hypercalciuria, and hypergammaglobulinemia are prevalent.

Sarcoidosis is a diagnosis of exclusion. A positive BAL shows an increased number of lymphocytes, with a helper/suppressor ratio of > 4:1 (hypersensitivity pneumonitis has a ratio of < 1). It is imperative to exclude the other granulomatous diseases, including hypersensitivity pneumonitis, berylliosis, and infectious diseases caused by mycobacteria and fungi. Material for histological exam should be cultured, as well as examined for organisms. While ensuring no organisms are present and cultures are negative, fiberoptic bronchoscopy with transbronchial or bronchial wall biopsies showing noncaseating granuloma are the best method for diagnosis of sarcoidosis.

Erythema nodosum is an associated skin lesion that denotes a good prognosis!

Treatment: Overall, 75% of sarcoid patients recover without treatment. It rarely progresses to pulmonary fibrosis or pulmonary hypertension. Treat severe disease with corticosteroids, for lack of anything better. There is no set regimen. Corticosteroids have not been proven to induce remissions in sarcoidosis, although they do decrease the symptoms, and PFTs improve. Inhaled corticosteroids decrease the respiratory symptoms and may be used instead of systemic corticosteroids if the disease is primarily in the bronchi. Indication for systemic corticosteroids is involvement of other organs: eyes, heart conduction abnormalities, CNS, severe pulmonary symptoms, severe skin lesions, and persistent hypercalcemia. Other medications available include hydroxychloroquine (Plaquenil®), infliximab (Remicade®), methotrexate, and thalidomide.

Eosinophilic Granuloma

Eosinophilic granuloma is also called Langerhans cell granulomatosis. It was previously called "Histiocytosis X." Virtually all affected patients are smokers and M > F. Langerhans cells are the predominant cell form. Patients have an interstitial disease with normal or increased lung volume (most IPFs have decreased lung volume). The granuloma can cause lytic bone lesions. It sometimes involves the posterior pituitary—leading to diabetes insipidus. In the lung, it causes interstitial changes and small cystic spaces in the upper lung fields, both of which are visible on chest x-ray, giving a "honeycomb appearance" (buzzword). Eosinophilic granulomatosis causing the combination of lytic bone lesions, diabetes insipidus, and exophthalmus is called Hand-Schüller-Christian syndrome.

10% of patients initially present with a pneumothorax, and up to 50% of these patients get a pneumothorax some time in the course of their illness.

Diagnose by finding Langerhans cells on lung biopsy or BAL.

Treatment of eosinophilic granuloma: Stop smoking! Many do a trial of steroids, although drugs generally do not help. Occasionally, there is spontaneous resolution. Again: Eosinophilic granuloma: pneumothorax, smoking.

Lymphangioleiomyomatosis

Lymphangioleiomyomatosis (LAM) occurs almost exclusively in premenopausal women. It is the result of immature smooth muscle proliferation in the lymphatic, vascular, and alveolar wall/peribronchial structures. This proliferation results in the formation of constrictions and cysts in these structures. There is a genetic relationship to tuberous sclerosis. Chest x-ray in LAM typically shows honeycombing (small cystic spaces) spread diffusely throughout the lung (in contrast to upper lung fields seen in eosinophilic granuloma above). Thoracic and abdominal lymphatics are often involved,

Table 3-4: Sarcoidosis Staging	
Radiographic Staging of Sarcoidosis	
STAGE	Chest X-ray Findings
0	Clear
I	Bilateral hilar adenopathy
II	Adenopathy + parenchymal infiltrates
III	Diffuse parenchymal infiltrates
IV	Fibrosis, bullae, cavities

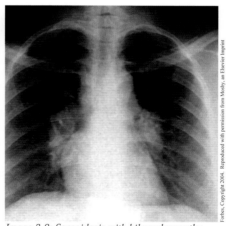

Image 3-8: Sarcoidosis with hilar adenopathy

Forbes, Copyright 2004. Reproduced with permission from Mosby, an Elsevier Imprint

notes

resulting in chylous pleural effusions—with triglycerides > 110 mg/dL +/– chylomicrons in the fluid. Pneumothorax may occur. Stop exogenous estrogens. Treatment is lung transplantation, but the process may recur in the transplanted lung.

Again: LAM: premenopausal, pneumothorax, chylous effusion (TG > 110 +/– chylomicrons), and associated with tuberous sclerosis.

Vasculitides that Cause ILD

Wegener Granulomatosis and ILD

Wegener granulomatosis—"necrotizing granuloma" (buzzword) is a vasculitis that:
1) affects the upper respiratory tract and paranasal sinuses
2) causes a granulomatous pulmonary vasculitis with large (sometimes cavitary) nodules
3) causes a necrotizing glomerulonephritis

It sometimes is limited just to the lungs (called "limited" Wegener's)

The ANCA test (antineutrophil cytoplasmic antibody—thought to be a destructive autoantibody) is often used as an adjunctive test. It is ~ 90% sensitive and 90% specific. When positive in a patient with Wegener's, it is virtually always c-ANCA (96%); polyarteritis is usually p-ANCA-positive.

Confirm diagnosis from either a biopsy of the nasal membrane or an open lung biopsy. A kidney biopsy is not part of the diagnostic workup, because it may not show the granulomas and is much more invasive. Treatment of Wegener granulomatosis: cyclophosphamide +/- corticosteroids.

Remember: Kidney, lungs, and sinuses. Consider Wegener's in any patient who presents with a purulent nasal discharge, epistaxis, and/or signs of a glomerulonephritis with hematuria. The patient is not dyspneic, and may or may not have a nonproductive cough or hemoptysis. If dyspneic and ANCA-negative, think Goodpasture syndrome.

Lymphomatoid Granulomatosis

Lymphomatoid granulomatosis—50% progress to histiocytic lymphoma. It is similar to Wegener's, but has no upper respiratory lesions and only rarely affects the kidney. Although the principal site is the lungs, lymphomatoid granulomatosis less often has skin, CNS, and peripheral nerve involvement. Biopsy shows a mononuclear angiocentric necrotic vasculitis. It is usually treated with corticosteroids and cyclophosphamide.

Allergic Granulomatosis of Churg-Strauss

Allergic granulomatosis of Churg-Strauss is a necrotizing, small-vessel vasculitis with eosinophilic infiltration. It may affect the skin and kidney, and may cause neuropathy. It does not affect the sinuses. Patients usually present with preexisting asthma and have eosinophilia (up to 80% of the WBCs). Consider this disease when assessing a progressively worsening asthmatic (along with ABPA).

Churg-Strauss may be unmasked by treating the asthmatic patient with a leukotriene-receptor antagonist and no corticosteroid preparation.

Treatment of Churg-Strauss: Aggressive therapy with cytotoxic agents and corticosteroids.

Bronchocentric Granulomatosis

Bronchocentric granulomatosis causes an ILD in which there are masses of granulomata in the walls and surrounding tissues of airways.

Polyarteritis Nodosa

Polyarteritis nodosa is the only one of this group that is not granulomatous. It is a necrotizing nongranulomatous vasculitis of medium-size arteries. "Painful Purple Papules" (buzz phrase). As noted above, polyarteritis nodosa is usually p-ANCA–positive (Polyarteritis: Painful Purple Papules, P-ANCA Positive) More on PAN in the Rheumatology section.

Eosinophilic ILDs

Overview

The eosinophilic ILDs are eosinophilic pneumonia, ABPA, and Churg-Strauss syndrome (the last discussed previously). Remember that asthma, hypereosinophilic syndrome, certain parasite infections, and some drugs are non-ILD causes of peripheral eosinophilia.

Eosinophilic Pneumonia

Eosinophilic pneumonia consists of 3 types:
1) Acute, benign eosinophilic pneumonia: Loeffler syndrome. Usually found incidentally. Minimal respiratory symptoms. These patients have migratory peripheral infiltrates on chest x-ray. Eosinophils are in the blood and sputum. In this and the other cases, you must rule out drugs and parasites.
2) Acute eosinophilic pneumonia: An acute, febrile, pulmonary illness with hypoxemic respiratory failure resembling ARDS. Unknown cause. Rule out infection. Treatment is ventilatory support and systemic corticosteroids.
3) Chronic eosinophilic pneumonia: The most common eosinophilic pneumonia in the U.S., and it usually occurs in middle-aged women. The illness is subacute with cough, wheezing, night sweats, and low-grade fever. 50% have a history of asthma. The chest x-ray shows bilateral, very peripheral infiltrates in a pattern that is the photographic negative of pulmonary edema (instead of a butterfly pattern of whiteness, the chest x-ray butterfly pattern looks dark). High eosinophils in the BAL, but 1/3 have no peripheral eosinophils. Very high ESR. Treatment is long-term steroids; relapses are common.

Acute Bronchopulmonary Aspergillosis (ABPA)

More on acute bronchopulmonary aspergillosis (ABPA): Caused by an allergic reaction to *Aspergillus*, in which there is immune-complex deposition. There is usually a very high

notes

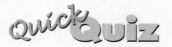

Quick Quiz

1) What is the treatment of c-ANCA-positive vasculitis that involves the lungs, sinuses, and kidneys?

2) Which vasculitis commonly progresses to histiocytic lymphoma?

3) An asthma patient with worsening symptoms and an eosinophil count of 75% makes you think of what diseases?

4) What presents on CXR as the "photographic negative" of CHF?

5) A "fingers-in-glove" pattern on chest CT should make you think of what disease? What is a common presentation of this disease?

6) What 2 organ systems does Goodpasture syndrome mainly affect?

serum IgE. The allergic reaction causes Type I (immediate wheal and flare; IgE-mediated) and Type III (5 hours), but not Type IV (delayed) reactions. Suspect it in asthmatics with worsening asthma symptoms, coughing brownish mucous plugs (!), recurrent infiltrates, and peripheral eosinophilia. ABPA may occur in CF patients.

Chest x-ray and CT show central mucous impaction and central bronchiectasis causing a "fingers-in-glove" appearing central infiltrate. Sputum may show branching hyphae (nonspecific). If there is only lung eosinophilia (no peripheral eos), think of a chronic eosinophilic pneumonia instead (see above).

Treatment of active ABPA (i.e., not in remission and not fibrotic) is long-term corticosteroids. Itraconazole is added if there is a poor or slow response to the corticosteroids.

Alveolar Proteinosis

Alveolar proteinosis—this disease is usually more alveolar than interstitial. There are defective alveolar macrophages causing a buildup of pulmonary surfactant. Symptoms are similar to those in silicosis, but there is no history of exposure to silica. Often, patients are hypoxemic from a large R-to-L shunt. Diagnosis is usually confirmed with open lung biopsy, but transbronchial biopsy or BAL is also okay. Treatment: If severe, do a whole lung lavage under general anesthesia. GM-CSF is a treatment that may restore proper function to the alveolar macrophages.

Idiopathic Pulmonary Hemosiderosis

Idiopathic pulmonary hemosiderosis causes intermittent pulmonary hemorrhage. DLCO can be elevated. It is similar to Goodpasture (below), except IPH does not affect the kidneys. Macrophages are filled with hemosiderin. Fe deficiency anemia occurs. It may remit in young patients, but it is unrelenting in adults. Remember that pulmonary hemorrhage also occurs in SLE.

Goodpasture Syndrome

Goodpasture syndrome has an autoimmune etiology. Usually young adult males; M to F is 3:1. Lung disease is the same as IPH (above), but Goodpasture syndrome also affects the kidneys. Usually, there is no frank hemorrhage, but often there is hemoptysis that precedes renal abnormalities. Like patients with IPH, these patients also may have Fe deficiency anemia. Symptoms are due to anti-glomerular, basement membrane antibodies that result in linear deposition of IgG and C3 on alveolar and glomerular BM. Treat with immunosuppressives and plasmapheresis. If the patient does have severe pulmonary hemorrhages, nephrectomy may help. Think of this disease if the patient presents with dyspnea, hemoptysis, Fe deficiency anemia, and glomerulonephritis—but without upper airway signs (Wegener's).

DIAGNOSIS OF ILDS

PFTs in ILD patients classically show a "restrictive intrathoracic" pattern. This means normal airway flow rates, but FVCs are low. There is increased lung stiffness (i.e., increased elastic recoil). A chest x-ray with diffuse interstitial infiltrates is often the first suggestion of disease, but it correlates poorly with severity of disease. The newer, high resolution CT scans (HRCT; with 1–2 mm cuts) are very useful in the workup of ILD.

Some x-ray clues of the cause of ILD:
- asbestosis: lower lung field predominance of infiltrates +/– pleural calcifications and plaques
- silicosis: hilar eggshell calcifications
- sarcoidosis: bilateral symmetrical hilar and paratracheal lymphadenopathy
- lymphangioleiomyomatosis (LAM): ILD with a pneumothorax in a premenopausal woman. May also have chylous effusions and characteristic nodules and cysts on CT

Bronchoscopy with transbronchial biopsy is the usual method for confirming the diagnosis and establishing the etiology and severity of ILD. However, the tissue specimens are small, and the best use of this technique is to diagnose and rule out:
- diffuse infections
- diffuse lymphangitic spread of carcinoma
- sarcoidosis

Thoracoscopic biopsy (through the chest wall) and open lung biopsy generally give the best yield for interstitial pneumonitis.

PULMONARY HEMORRHAGE

Causes of diffuse alveolar hemorrhage and/or pulmonary hemorrhage:
- Bronchitis
- Tuberculosis
- Severe thrombocytopenia
- Bronchiectasis
- Lung abscess
- Aspergilloma

notes

- Aspergillosis, mucormycosis, and other acute fungal infections
- Chemotherapy and bone marrow transplantation

Immunologic lung diseases that cause pulmonary hemorrhage:
- Goodpasture syndrome
- SLE
- Wegener granulomatosis
- IPH

Cardiopulmonary diseases that cause pulmonary hemorrhage:
- Pulmonary AV malformations
- Aortic aneurysm
- Pulmonary hypertension
- Septic R heart emboli
- Mitral stenosis

PULMONARY HYPERTENSION

Primary pulmonary hypertension (PPH) is an idiopathic process, typically occurring in young women, that eventually causes easy fatigability, syncope, and chest pain and dyspnea on exertion. PPH affects entire vasculature of the lung, including the endothelium, smooth muscle, and even the extracellular matrix. This results in an obliterative process in which the pulmonary vessels become more torturous and close off. Persons with Raynaud disease are more likely to get PPH. In making the diagnosis of PPH, you must exclude potentially treatable causes of increased pulmonary artery pressure (i.e., all $2°$ causes).

Secondary pulmonary hypertension can be caused by diseases that increase resistance to blood flow in the lung. SPH can be caused by chronic hypoxia (the most potent stimulus for vasoconstriction—e.g., severe COPD, severe sleep apnea), polycythemia vera (PCV), chronic or multiple pulmonary emboli, and any of the parenchymal lung diseases. Remember that scleroderma causes pulmonary hypertension out of proportion to the apparent pulmonary disease, because the pulmonary manifestation in scleroderma is intimal proliferation. Outside of the U.S., think of filariasis and schistosomiasis or mitral stenosis/valvular heart diseases as possible causes.

Physical exam: Loud 2nd heart sound (P_2), tricuspid regurgitation, RV heave.

Best diagnostic test for pulmonary hypertension is right heart catheterization, in which pulmonary artery diastolic pressure (PADP) > PCWP and usually > 20 mmHg and there is elevated RA pressure.

Echocardiograms also assist with diagnosis and management because they:
- can estimate pulmonary artery pressure
- evaluate right ventricular size, wall thickness, and systolic motion
- evaluate right atrial size
- evaluate the presence of a R-to-L shunt through a patent foramen ovale (need echo contrast agent for shunt detection)

ECG may show right axis deviation from RVH, while the chest x-ray exhibits engorged pulmonary arteries. Tricuspid regurgitation is common with pulmonary hypertension, and is due to the dilation of the right ventricle (holosystolic murmur along the LLSB—increases with inspiration—and a parasternal heave). The tricuspid regurgitation and right ventricular failure presents as JVD with large v waves, liver pulsations, and lower extremity edema.

Treatment of pulmonary hypertension [Know!]:

Bosentan (Tracleer®) is an oral endothelin antagonist—a polypeptide that is released by injured endothelium. It is elevated in patients with PH and heart failure.

The pulmonary vasodilators of choice are the calcium channel blockers—especially nifedipine, amlodipine, and diltiazem. Amlodipine especially if intolerant of other calcium-channel blockers, and diltiazem especially if tachycardic.

Short-acting pulmonary vasodilators, such as inhaled nitric oxide and IV adenosine, have only a transient effect. Use these while hemodynamically monitoring the patient. Inhaled iloprost, an inhaled vasodilator, helps with symptoms, but improvement in survival has not been demonstrated.

Continuous IV (pump) infusion of epoprostenol (prostacyclin) has now been approved for treatment of functional class III and IV patients who are unresponsive to other treatments, and have demonstrated good results with prostacyclin. However, these patients exhibit tachyphylaxis and require slow "ramp-up" of the dosing over time.

Sildenafil (Revatio™) inhibits cyclic guanosine monophosphate (cGMP) phosphodiesterase type 5 (PDE-5) in smooth muscle of pulmonary vasculature, where PDE-5 is responsible for the degradation of cGMP. Increased cGMP concentration results in pulmonary vasculature relaxation, and vasodilation in the pulmonary bed may occur.

Give anticoagulants to prevent thrombosis and pulmonary emboli.

Oxygen helps symptoms in PH secondary to COPD. Give oxygen to all who meet the criteria as discussed in COPD (see pg 3-13). Occasionally, single lung transplantation or heart-lung transplantation are long-term solutions.

VENOUS THROMBOEMBOLISM (VTE)
OVERVIEW

Venous thromboembolism (VTE) is the term that includes both deep venous thromboses (DVTs) and pulmonary emboli (PEs). DVTs and PEs are considered the same disease process; the majority of medically significant pulmonary emboli are from DVTs in lower extremities—virtually all from above the knee (ileofemoral area). Most DVTs occurring below the knee do not embolize.

Other sources of PEs are upper extremity, internal jugular, and subclavian thrombi. Especially consider these areas if an IV catheter is in place.

Pulmonary embolism is the 3rd most common cardiovascular cause of death (after ischemic heart disease and stroke); 11% die within 1 hour of onset of symptoms. Despite our knowledge of the cause and effect of PEs, the incidence has not declined. In hospitalized patients, inadequate VTE prophylaxis is the usual cause.

notes

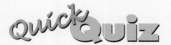

Quick Quiz

1) In what group does primary pulmonary hypertension occur?
2) What is the best test to diagnose pulmonary hypertension?
3) From where do most pulmonary emboli arise?
4) A catheter in a large vein in the upper extremity increases the risk of _____?

Sequence of events in a medically significant PE: embolic obstruction of a pulmonary artery is followed by:
- increased alveolar dead space—ventilated but not perfused
- vascular constriction
- loss of alveolar surfactant with atelectasis—V/Q mismatch + shunt areas

This results in an increased resistance to blood flow → increased pulmonary artery pressure → increased right ventricular work. Because of increased capacitance of the pulmonary circulation, usually up to 50% of the lung vasculature can be blocked before increased workload on the right ventricle becomes significant. Massive PE occurs when > 2/3 of a lung is involved.

Note that lung-tissue infarction is rare (< 10%) because the tissue is fed by multiple sources, including the bronchial artery, the PA, and back-diffusion through the pulmonary venous system.

CLINICAL FINDINGS IN PE

Overview

First we will go over the clinical findings and tests. Then we will go through a systematic evidence-based workup of PE.

Clinical findings are varied and usually nonspecific, but there is a suggestive set of signs and symptoms. Sudden onset of dyspnea and tachypnea are most common. Hemoptysis and pleurisy indicate associated lung infarction.

Pleurisy and friction rubs are actually seen more often in submassive PE, because they are due to a distal impaction of the vessel; and so they occur nearer to the pleura, in which case these symptoms are probably due to more a local inflammatory reaction than lung infarction.

Clinical Findings

There is a combination of 3 clinical findings that is more specific for a massive PE:
1) increased P_2 (pulmonic heart sound),
2) S_3 and/or S_4 gallop, and
3) cyanosis.

A massive PE has characteristic findings on right heart catheterization (Swan-Ganz). As the catheter is being positioned, you would see an elevated RA pressure. Once the catheter is placed, pulmonary artery diastolic pressure (PADP) is greater than the PCWP. Increased pulmonary vascular resistance is indicated by this elevated PADP-PCWP gradient.

Note: The Wells prediction rules for DVT (Table 3-5) and for PE (Table 3-6) determine the pretest probability of DVT and/or PE, and doing these (or similar verified pretest probability rules) is the first step of the diagnostic workup for VTE (Figure 3-7).

Review of Lab and Radiological Tests

There are 9 techniques used in the evaluation of possible PE. First I'll list them, and then we'll discuss each one [Know all of them!]:

1) ABGs	2) chest x-rays
3) ECG	4) V/Q scan
5) venous studies	6) pulmonary angiography
7) MDCT	8) MRI/MRA

9) transthoracic or transesophageal echocardiography

1) ABGs indicate hypoxia, necessitating further inquiry. Analysis of data from the Prospective Investigation of Pulmonary Embolism Diagnosis (PIOPED) indicates that neither ABGs nor A-a gradient is useful in the diagnosis or triaging of patients with pulmonary embolism. An A-a O_2 difference ($D_{A-a}O_2$) > 20 mmHg is seen in 89% of patients with a PE. Inversely, only 11% of those with a PE have a $D_{A-a}O_2 < 20$ mmHg. Only in the absence of cardiopulmonary disease and if the patient is not on O_2 and is not hyperventilating is the size of the embolus reflected by the decrease in P_aO_2!

Hypoxemia, after a large PE, is due to many factors—especially V/Q mismatch, R-to-L shunt, and dead space—although dead space must be very large to cause hypoxia. The V/Q mismatch is from decreased perfusion of ventilated areas. The shunt is from perfusion of poorly ventilated areas that occur as a side effect of PE ($2°$ to broncho-constrictive mediators and atelectasis). Secondary right ventricular failure can also contribute to the V/Q mismatch.

2) Chest x-ray helps rule out other causes in the differential (pneumonia, pneumothorax). Chest x-ray findings are common but pretty nonspecific in PE: infiltrate, effusion, atelectasis; and 12% have no x-ray abnormalities. Even so, a PE is suggested by:
- near-normal or normal chest x-ray in a dyspneic patient
- pulmonary infiltrate with a normal WBC count on peripheral smear

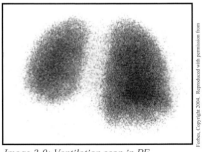
Image 3-9: Ventilation scan in PE

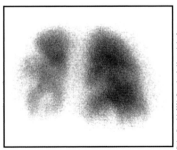
Image 3-10: Perfusion scan in PE

notes

- pulmonary consolidation associated with an elevated ipsilateral hemidiaphragm (from atelectasis)
- "Hampton hump"—a pleural-based, wedge-shape defect from infarction just above the diaphragm
- Oligemia (Westermark sign; rarely seen)—a lack of vascular markings in the area downstream of the embolus
- Large right descending pulmonary artery

Remember: The most common chest x-ray finding in a PE is nothing (i.e., a normal chest x-ray)!

3) ECG. The only specific (but not sensitive) heart/ECG changes seen with PE are tachycardia and right ventricle strain (i.e., acute cor pulmonale). On ECG, right heart strain = S_1-Q_3-T_3; that is, the S wave is large in I, the Q wave is large in III, and the T wave is inverted in III. This is not seen much, but it is worth checking. ECG also helps rule out an MI.

4) Ventilation/Perfusion lung scan is one of the most widely used diagnostic tests for PE.
- Normal: A normal chest x-ray plus a normal perfusion study is associated with a very low risk of PE. When coupled with a low clinical probability for PE, a normal chest x-ray can substitute for the ventilation scan! Even so, you usually order the ventilation and perfusion scans at the same time. When coupled with a low clinical probability, a normal V/Q scan eliminates the diagnosis of PE.
- Low-probability and moderate-probability scans are considered indeterminate, because these patients have 14–40% chance of PE.
- Moderate-probability scans consist of subsegmental perfusion defects or matched ventilation and perfusion defects. A chest x-ray finding of an infiltrate in the area of perfusion defect indicates the same risk. If clinical suspicion of PE is low, no further testing is necessary. If it is high, do a pulmonary arteriogram or leg studies. Remember, if you suspect a PE, start heparin before the patient goes for the V/Q scan.
- High-probability scans occur when:
  a) $\geq$ 2 segmental or larger perfusion defects are present with a normal ventilation study, or
  b) the perfusion defect is much larger than the ventilation defect.

The trouble with V/Q scans is that large numbers come back as low-probability/indeterminate. You greatly improve accuracy of the above scans by factoring in clinical suspicion or clinical probability of a PE. For instance:
- ~ 30% of patients with a low-probability scan have a PE, but with a low clinical probability, this rate drops to 2%! And with a high clinical probability, it jumps to 40%.
- ~ 85% of patients with a high-probability scan have a PE, but with a high clinical probability, this rate jumps to 96%! And with a low clinical probability, it plummets to 6%.

Determining the probability for PE (by means of a verified test) is included as the first step of the diagnostic workup.

5) Venous studies. PE and DVT (deep venous thrombosis) are 2 manifestations of the same disease process. Determining the existence of DVT of the lower extremities can be an important adjunct in diagnosing and preventing a PE. The presence of DVT mandates treatment with anticoagulants, unless there are contraindications.

Another point: Determining lower extremities as the probable source is also important because inferior vena caval interruption may be necessary to treat emboli that occur while adequately anticoagulated, or in a setting where contraindications prevent you from anticoagulating the patient.

Although few DVTs of calf origin actually do migrate above the knee, the ones that do are usually painful! So you would usually place a patient with a painful calf DVT on anticoagulants. If a patient has a painless calf DVT, follow up with serial ultrasound studies.

The contrast venogram (ascending phlebography) is still the gold standard for verifying DVT of the lower extremities. It is the only test reliable for any asymptomatic patient in whom DVT is suspected. Because of vessel abnormalities commonly found in persons previously treated for DVT, contrast venogram is also the best test for diagnosing recurrent DVT.

Impedance plethysmography (IPG) is a sensitive, noninvasive test. Operator-dependent. Sensitivity and specificity are good only in symptomatic patients being evaluated for their first DVT. You can use IPG for recurrent DVT if the IPG returned to normal after the first DVT.

Duplex ultrasonography combines real-time, B-mode ultrasonography, which visualizes the vessel with Doppler flow detection. Also operator-dependent. Like IPG, venous ultrasonography is reliable only in symptomatic patients being evaluated for their first DVT. In these patients, the sensitivity is 93% with a 98% specificity. It is poor for detecting distal DVT (because the vessels are hard to visualize).

Note: Malignancy is present in 50% of patients with phlegmasia cerulea dolens. Malignancy is also suggested by superficial migratory thrombophlebitis, DVT resistant to anticoagulants, and thrombophlebitis in unusual places such as the arms and trunk. Also, DVT in a young person with no risk factors indicates a 19 x normal possibility of underlying malignancy!

CT scan is better than any of the previous tests (including contrast venography) for detecting thrombosed vessels in the abdomen and pelvis. Also see multidetector CT (#7 below). Some centers combine CT of legs and pelvis with the PE protocol—contrast-enhanced CT to look for PE and DVT simultaneously.

MRI appears to be the best (but most expensive) noninvasive test available for determining DVT of the proximal vessels. It is 100% sensitive and 97% specific.

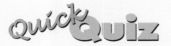
D-dimer testing has become more sensitive and more useful—used with any one of the above noninvasive tests, it increases the negative predictive value of the test. A negative D-dimer, along with a low pretest probability in a younger patient with negative history of VTE and no comorbidity has a 96–99% negative predictive value for VTE (DVT and/or PE). A negative D-dimer with a negative IPG has a 99% negative predictive value for VTE. In either of these cases, VTE is ruled out.

Note: Use the more sensitive ELISA, quantitative rapid ELISA, or turbidimetric D-dimer assays (not latex agglutination).

Because of the lack of specificity, the D-dimer has a poor positive predictive value, so it is not used alone to screen for DVT.

6) Pulmonary angiography is the gold standard for diagnosis of PE. Because it is an invasive test, it is reserved for cases with unsatisfactory results from previous tests. Do not use pulmonary angiography if there is:
- a high probability V/Q scan, or
- evidence of DVT

Pulmonary angiography is indicated for patients with suggestive symptoms or high pretest probability of PE with indeterminate (or low probability) V/Q scans or MDCT (below), and a negative DVT workup. Pulmonary angiography, especially if selective (guided by V/Q or MDCT scan findings), is a relatively safe procedure. Mortality < 0.1%, morbidity = 1-2%.

7) Multidetector CT (MDCT) is the next generation of helical CT (previously, it was single-detector helical CT). It allows 1.2 mm sections during a single held breath. MDCT also evaluates for other diagnoses that could mimic a PE. It is now often used in place of a V/Q scan when the patient has cardiopulmonary problems that might obscure the results of the V/Q scan.

8) MRI/MRA. MRI alone is showing good potential in visualization of the pulmonary vessels. Evaluation is in progress. Magnetic resonance angiography (MRA) is another, newer test with promise. It can view up to 8th-order vessels. It is not available on all MRI machines.

9) Transthoracic and transesophageal echo have poor sensitivity and specificity, and are not indicated for the diagnosis of PE. They are useful in determining right ventricular strain/overload during PE workup. You may see clots in the central vessels with TEE, but it is not recommended as the main test.

Diagnosis of VTE

So, how is the diagnosis of VTE made?
1) Use clinical prediction rules (Wells most commonly cited) to determine pretest probability of DVT and/or PE. See Table 3-5 and Table 3-6.
2) In patients with low pretest probability, a negative highly sensitive D-dimer indicates a low likelihood of venous thromboembolism and excludes the diagnosis.
3) U/S of lower extremities is recommended for patients with intermediate-to-high pretest probability of DVT.
4) Patients with intermediate or high pretest probability of PE require imaging studies (V/Q scan, multidetector helical CT, or pulmonary angiography).

See Figure 3-7 for a flowchart of the full workup.

Venous studies have not been fully evaluated on patients with cardiopulmonary disease, so do a pulmonary angiogram along with venous studies (yeah, do them anyway) instead on

Table 3-5: Wells Criteria for DVT	
CRITERIA	Score
Active cancer (Current tx or palliation, or tx within last 6 mo)	1
Recent immobilization of lower extremities (plaster cast, paralysis, paresis)	1
Recently bedridden > 3 days or major surgery with general/regional anesthesia	1
Localized tenderness along the distribution of deep venous system	1
Entire leg swollen	1
Calf swelling 3 cm larger than asymptomatic side (measured 10 cm below tibial tuberosity)	1
Pitting edema confined to the symptomatic leg	1
Collateral nonvaricose superficial veins	1
Alternative diagnosis is at least as likely as DVT	-2
3 or higher = high probability of DVT 1-2 = moderate probability 0 = low probability	
Note: if symptoms are in both legs, use the more symptomatic one.	

notes

Table 3-6: Wells Criteria for PE

CRITERIA	Points
Clinical signs of DVT	3.0
An alternative diagnosis is LESS likely than PE	3.0
Heart rate >100 beats/min	1.5
Immobilization or surgery in the previous 4 wks	1.5
Previous DVT/PE	1.5
Hemoptysis	1.0
Malignancy (being treated, treated in the past 6 mo, or palliative)	1.0

0-1 = Low probability of PE
2-6 = Moderate probability
> 6 = High probability

TREATMENT OF PE

Adjunctive Treatment

Give oxygen for hypoxia. Many use dobutamine for right heart failure, because it has both inotropic and pulmonary vasodilating effects.

Anticoagulants

Overview

Achieve adequate anticoagulation ASAP! Anticoagulants are indicated for PE and DVT—unless there are absolute contraindications, which are discussed below.

The anticoagulant treatment options for PE are IV unfractionated heparin (UH) or subcutaneous low molecular weight heparin (LMWH) for 7–10 days, followed by LMWH or warfarin for 3–6 months for VTE due to transient risk factors, 12 months for idiopathic VTE, and indefinitely for recurrent VTEs.

Now we'll discuss the various anticoagulants and in which cases we use which one!

these patients. Optionally, you can do a MDCT instead of V/Q scan on these patients.

Fat emboli cause the triad of dyspnea, confusion, and petechiae—usually in the neck, axilla, and/or conjunctiva. You do not need a V/Q scan for diagnosis if this triad is present! Fat emboli occur within 72 hours after a fracture of a large bone (e.g., femur), sometimes after CPR, and with sickle cell bone-occlusive crisis. Treatment is supportive; unless the patient has secondary ARDS, corticosteroids have not proven helpful.

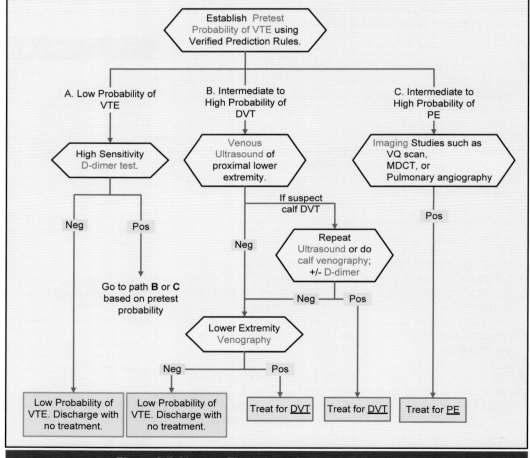

Figure 3-7: Venous Thromboembolism (VTE) Workup

notes

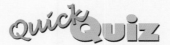

Note. Do not give anticoagulants to patients with:
- uncorrected major bleeding disorder (thrombocytopenia, hemophilias, liver failure, renal failure)
- uncontrolled severe hypertension (systolic > 200 mmHg, diastolic > 140 mmHg)
- potential bleeding lesions (active peptic ulcer, esophageal varices, aneurysm, recent trauma or surgery to head/orbit/spine, recent stroke, intracranial or intraspinal bleed)
- using NSAIDs—increases GI bleed—if able, stop NSAIDs
- having repeated falls or unstable gait
- protein C deficiency (risk of skin necrosis)
- or to uncooperative/unreliable patients

Heparin

Unfractionated heparin (UH) binds with antithrombin (AT) to make it 1000–4000x more effective in inactivating thrombin and factor Xa. To inactivate the thrombin, heparin binds to both the AT and the thrombin.

Unfractionated heparin is no longer the drug of choice for DVT, but it is still used for initial treatment of PE. Low molecular weight heparin (LMWH; discussed below) is the drug of choice now for DVT and is at least as good as UH for PE.

UH dosage is determined by means of a weight-based nomogram to achieve adequate anticoagulation. Do PTT levels every 6–8 hours after dosage change (to allow time to achieve steady state).

Adjust the dose of IV UH to keep the PTT at least 1.5 x control for 7–10 days. Then continue anticoagulant treatment as discussed above (minimum 3–6 months), preferably with either LMWH based on body weight or warfarin (see below). Adjusted-dose heparin is used by some—dosing to maintain PTT at 1.5 x control. Greater increases than these result in increased incidence of bleeding.

Complications: The major problem with UH use is hemorrhage. Before giving it, be sure the patient has no major bleeding syndrome, no recent bleed, and has heme-negative stool. Heparin-induced thrombocytopenia (HIT) is common and usually of no clinical consequence, but always monitor platelet count and stop using heparin (even heparin flushes) if platelet count drops > 50%, and check heparin antibodies.

LMWH: Subcutaneous full-dose LMWH (tinzaparin, reviparin, dalteparin, nadroparin, and enoxaparin) should be used whenever possible for DVT (lower risk of major bleeding compared to UH). Either LMWH or UH can be used for initial treatment of PE—LMWH is preferred by most.

LMWH is made from the depolymerization of heparin, which produces some molecular fragments with 30–50% the weight and more anticoagulant activity. LMWH has no effect on thrombin like heparin does—rather it solely inactivates factor Xa. It has been proven to cause fewer instances of major bleed than UH in DVT (studies pending for PE), and anticoagulation is established more quickly than with UH in any VTE situation. Also, much lower incidence of HIT.

LMWH is recommended (per ACCP) as an alternative to UH for treating VTE in pregnant women. If necessary, you can monitor activity by assessing activated factor Xa levels.

LMWH is the recommended treatment of VTE for cancer patients.

LMWH is used for outpatient treatment of DVT and even PE in certain lower-risk and carefully followed patients.

Do not monitor the PTT in patients on LMWH, because LMWH does not affect thrombin and therefore has no effect on PTT (solely on activated factor Xa). LMWH still causes heparin-induced thrombocytopenia (although less than UH), so monitor platelet count.

Warfarin

Note: "International normalized ratio" (INR) is a product of the $PT_{patient}/PT_{control}$ ratio times an "international sensitivity index" (ISI). The ISI accounts for the sensitivity of the thromboplastin used by the lab, which varies from batch to batch. The formula is $INR = (PT_{patient}/PT_{control}) \times ISI$. INR is the test to determine proper dosing of warfarin.

Warfarin is a vitamin K antagonist that prevents activation of factors II, VII, IX, and X. Absolute contraindications include pregnancy. Remember: After starting warfarin, factor VII is the most rapidly decreasing procoagulant, but protein C (an anticoagulant) also decreases rapidly—so you may rarely see an initial net procoagulant effect, even though PT increases. This may occur only until the slower-clearing factor II decreases enough to result in a net anticoagulant state. This usually takes ~ 4 days. This potential problem is addressed by starting the warfarin right after heparin is started (within 8 hours), and keeping patients on heparin for at least 4 days.

Warfarin is adjusted to increase INR to 2.0–3.0. Initial dose is usually 5.0 mg/day, and this is often decreased to ~ 2.5 mg/day. This recommended starting dose of 5.0 mg is lower than that previously used—to avoid bleeding complications

notes

and paradoxical increase in clotting from protein C or S depletion (see above paragraph). It is usually given for 3–6 months. If DVT recurs just after stopping warfarin treatment, then resume anticoagulation for one year. Persons with permanent thrombotic tendencies (antithrombin III deficiency, protein C deficiency, lupus anticoagulant, or certain malignancies) should be anticoagulated for life.

Again, do not give warfarin to pregnant patients (deformities are common, especially if given in the first trimester). Use LMWH or adjusted-dose UH instead.

Warfarin necrosis is an idiosyncratic side effect of warfarin, which causes full-thickness skin necrosis requiring skin grafts.

Compression Stockings

Compression stockings are recommended for all patients with proximal DVT because they greatly decrease the incidence of post-thrombotic syndrome. Start within one month after DVT.

Thrombolytics

PE: Streptokinase, tPA, and other thrombolytics are now used to treat a significant acute PE with unstable hemodynamics not responding to treatment; e.g., when a patient with a PE "crashes."

Data support the use of thrombolytic therapy to treat patients with PE who have echocardiographic evidence of right ventricular overload, strain, or dysfunction secondary to the PE.

A more controversial use is to decrease long-term sequelae after a massive PE (obstruction of ≥ 2 segmental arteries or 1 lobar artery), and to give it within 5 days after onset of the PE—i.e., before the clot starts to organize. Thrombolytics appear to decrease the long-term sequelae of PE, such as chronic pulmonary hypertension.

Thrombolytics are now used to treat DVT and can maintain function of the valvular system and prevent post-phlebitis syndrome.

Surgery

Results from a study call into question the use of vena caval filters, such as the Greenfield filter. Current indications are to use these filters when there are recurring VTEs with adequate anticoagulation or when there are recurring VTEs, and anticoagulant treatment is contraindicated. A French study showed a negative benefit to placement in ill patients with DVT or PE. It resulted in a greater number of DVTs in a 2-year follow-up period. Despite this finding, an uncontested indication is when one of these patients has a pulmonary embolism and will die if another one occurs—e.g., if a patient has a massive PE after either a massive MI or heart surgery. Thrombectomy/embolectomy is a potential option but is associated with a high operative mortality rate.

RISK AND PROPHYLAXIS

Risk profile and prophylaxis [Know!]:

High Risk: Patients at highest risk for PE have an acute fracture of, or orthopedic procedure on, a lower extremity. Another high-risk procedure is extensive pelvic/abdominal surgery for cancer.

High-risk prophylaxis:
  • LMWH   • adjusted-dose heparin
  • warfarin (INR 2–3)   • dextran
  • external pneumatic compression (but not for lower extremity surgery!)

LMWH is often the prophylactic drug of choice for orthopedic surgery and nonhemorrhagic stroke.

Low-dose SQ heparin is not effective in the high-risk group. Remember that dextran can precipitate CHF in susceptible patients.

Moderate risk of PE is carried by any other surgery—including neurosurgery and trauma—especially in patients > 40 years old. Patients with CHF and those with pneumonias also have a moderate risk!

Moderate-risk prophylaxis:
  • external pneumatic compression (esp. neurosurgery)
  • low-dose SQ heparin 5000U SQ q 8h (previously was q 12h)

Lower but still significant risk includes all immobilized patients and those < age 40 undergoing thoracic or abdominal (including gynecologic) surgery.

Low-risk prophylaxis:
  • use graduated stockings and   • ensure early mobilization.

Acquired risk factors are lupus anticoagulant, nephrotic syndrome, and paroxysmal nocturnal hemoglobinuria (PNH).

Inherited risk factors (rare) are antithrombin III deficiency, protein C and S deficiencies, dysfibrinogenemia, and plasminogen problems. The most common inherited hypercoagulability disorder is resistance to activated protein C, an endogenous anticoagulant. This is caused by a point mutation, called factor V Leiden, in the factor V gene.

Pregnancy is a hypercoagulable state that lasts until 1–2 months after delivery; so aggressively treat pregnant women at risk for venous thromboembolism with subcutaneous adjusted-dose heparin, as needed, to maintain either PTT 1.5–2 x N or plasma heparin levels of 0.1–0.2 IU/ml. If this is not feasible, give heparin 7,500–10,000 IU SQ bid. In either case, switch to warfarin after delivery.

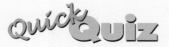

PLEURAL EFFUSIONS

Pleural effusions are either transudative or exudative.

A transudative effusion is a secondary phenomenon, due to systemic changes influencing the formation and absorption of pleural fluid. The most common causes are LV failure, pulmonary embolism, cirrhosis, and hydronephrosis.

An exudative effusion is due to a local cause; the most common causes are bacterial pneumonia, viral infection, malignancy, and pulmonary embolism.

	E/S protein		LDH$_{EFF}$		E/S LDH
Transudative:	< 0.5	*and*	< 200	*and*	< 0.6
Exudative:	> 0.5	*or*	> 200	*or*	> 0.6

Note that all 3 conditions must be met for an effusion to be called a transudate—failing any 1 criterion makes it an exudate.

Transudative effusions require no further workup, because they are reactive, systemic phenomena—treat the main problem.

Exudative effusions are associated with local disorders and require further tests on the fluid to establish the disorder.

Exudative effusion notes:

The most common causes of malignant pleural effusions are lung cancer (1/3), breast cancer (1/4), and lymphoma (1/5). Lung, breast, lymphoma...1/3, 1/4, 1/5. In a pleural-based malignancy, cytologic examination of the effusion fluid has as high a yield as pleural biopsy! 3 effusion samples have a combined yield of 90%.

Suspect "yellow nail syndrome" if the patient has a history of chronic peripheral edema and chronic exudative pleural effusions. Patients with this genetically transmitted syndrome will also have yellow, dystrophic nails.

Mesothelioma (considered pathognomonic of asbestos exposure) usually presents with a grossly hemorrhagic pleural effusion.

Bacteria in the effusion mean empyema, and a chest tube is usually required.

Transudative effusion notes:

You may see left-sided pleural effusion in association with pancreatitis.

Pleural effusions are common after abdominal surgery and usually benign.

Relief of dyspnea after therapeutic thoracentesis for an effusion is due to a decrease in intrathoracic volume!! This is because most of the volume a pleural effusion occupies is obtained by distending the diaphragm (which causes the dyspnea). Only about 20% of the volume is obtained from compression of the lung.

Workup of pleural effusion: On chest x-ray, effusions typically push the heart to the opposite side. If you see what appears to be an effusion and the heart is not shifted, consider atelectasis as the cause. If there is fluid, it is important to analyze it. The first differentiation to make is: Is it a transudate or exudate? An exudate is caused by an inflammatory condition and indicates the need for further workup.

Transudative or exudative? Upon draining the pleural fluid, check the appearance and test for protein and LDH in both the pleural fluid and the serum.

If the effusion is transudative, no further workup is needed; initiate treatment aimed at the systemic cause (CHF, kidney disease, cirrhosis). If the effusion is exudative, more lab tests are needed (on the tubes you saved!) to find the local cause—see below.

If the other lab work is normal, consider a V/Q lung scan or pulmonary angiogram to rule out pulmonary embolus, and a needle biopsy of the pleura to rule out cancer and tuberculosis. Also consider a chest CT to evaluate lung parenchyma, pleural surface, and subdiaphragmatic areas.

Parapneumonic effusions start out as sterile, reactive effusions precipitated by pneumonia. Timely treatment of the pneumonia with antibiotics prevents the progression of the effusion to an empyema. Without antibiotics, a loculated empyema can develop—even in as short a period as 1–2 days.

Some key effusion findings (not set in stone, just clues):

Cell count with differential findings:

WBCs > 1000, think exudate; > 10,000, think parapneumonic effusion (becoming an empyema); WBCs > 100,000 = empyema or pus.

Mesothelial cells normally line the cavity and are occasionally confused with malignant cells. These are rarely seen in a tuberculous effusion. So if results say no mesothelial cells, think tuberculous effusion.

Eosinophils > 10%: think pneumothorax, drug reaction, paragonimiasis (trematode: fluke), fungal infection, and asbestos exposure.

Lymphocytes > 50%: think TB or malignancy.

Neutrophil predominance: think pneumonia, pancreatitis, PE, peritonitis.

notes

Chemistry findings:

Glucose 80 = TB; 60 = cancer, empyema; < 30 = rheumatoid arthritis.

Amylase increased in pancreatic fistula, esophageal rupture (salivary amylase), or local malignancy (seen in 10% of malignant effusions).

pH is most useful in a parapneumonic effusion. In general, you see a low pH with malignancy, collagen-vascular disease, and granulomatous infection as cause of the effusion. A pH < 7.0 suggests complicated effusion (loculated) that may progress to empyema; pH < 7.2 suggests need for chest tube placement. Malignancy: pH < 7.3 in a malignant effusion suggests high tumor burden and poor likelihood of survival or successful pleurodesis.

Pleural fluid ANA > 1:160 in both drug-induced SLE and native SLE. If the ANA is positive, then check anti-dsDNA (specific for native SLE) and anti-histone (specific for drug-induced lupus).

Triglyceride level (on white samples—see next): > 115 mg/dl = chylous; < 50 = pseudochylous.

Chylous effusions are white-appearing, exudative effusions with a triglyceride level > 115 mg/dL (due to fat globules—i.e., chylomicrons). The chylous effusions are associated with leakage of thoracic duct lymph. This can be caused by trauma, lymphoma, mediastinal cancer/fibrosis, and lymphangioleiomyomatosis (LAM)!

Pseudochylous pleural effusions are associated with chronic inflammatory processes, especially TB and rheumatoid arthritis lung disease. Triglycerides in pseudochylous effusions are < 50 mg/dL, because the white color is due to cholesterol, not chylomicrons. Neither the chylous nor pseudochylous specimens clear with centrifugation.

If the cell count with differential suggests infection, get C&S and Gram stain. If you suspect malignancy, get cytology, glucose, and amylase.

Indications for a chest tube include:
• Pus in pleural space
• Positive culture on pleural space fluid
• Complicated parapneumonic effusion (i.e., loculated empyema)—most treat with antibiotics and drainage; some only tap and give antibiotics

If results are ambiguous, repeat the thoracentesis in 12–18 hours. If a loculated empyema does not respond quickly to chest tube and antibiotics, thoracotomy is indicated. Some pulmonary specialists recommend chest tube for complicated parapneumonic effusions. Streptokinase or urokinase can be instilled in complicated parapneumonic effusions and empyemas to enhance drainage and decrease the need for decortication surgery.

Always do a pleural biopsy if you suspect tuberculosis, because there is only a 20% sensitivity with the fluid cultures. With repeated biopsies, sensitivity increases to > 90%! Pleural biopsy works equally well with malignancy but so does effusion cytology. So biopsy is usually not done when malignancy is suspected. Closed pleural biopsy is rapidly being replaced by thorascopic biopsy procedure, because direct visu-

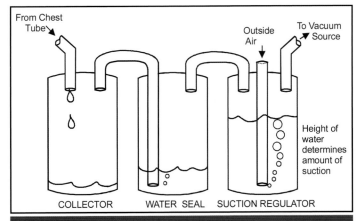

Figure 3-8: Pleurovac System

alization helps guide the biopsy. [Remember: pleural biopsy = TB; effusion cytology = cancer].

PNEUMOTHORAX

Primary, spontaneous pneumothorax (PSP) was once thought to be a benign problem that most commonly affects tall, slender, smoking men ages 20–40 years. With high-resolution CT, we now know that many of these patients have emphysematous blebs, which may be an etiologic factor.

Secondary spontaneous pneumothorax (SSP):
• COPD is the most common cause.
• PCP in AIDS patients occasionally causes a pneumothorax.

Other causes of SSP include:
• cystic fibrosis
• eosinophilic granuloma (histiocytosis X—smoking males)
• lymphangioleiomyomatosis (LAM—exclusively premenopausal women)
• About 10–15% of patients on mechanical ventilators develop barotrauma, including pneumothorax

Recurrence rate for PSP is 28%, while that for SSP is 43%. Risk of mortality is 1–4% for PSP and up to 17% for SSP.

Initial treatment:

If the pneumothorax is small (< 15–20%) and the patient is stable, observe the patient and give high-flow O_2. 3L/min O_2 by NC is associated with a 3-4–fold increase in rate of reabsorption (vs. room air). If the pneumothorax is larger, place a small anterior chest tube. This may consist of an intravenous catheter inserted via the 2nd intercostal space, aspirated, and either closed off or connected to suction. A chest tube is mandatory in pneumothorax patients receiving positive pressure ventilation!

A persistent air leak for > 7 days suggests a bronchopleural fistula, which may require surgical intervention for stapling and pleurodesis to prevent recurrences. Note: Some say corrective intervention should be done after 2 days; some say as long as 14 days.

notes

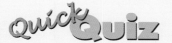

Quick Quiz

Review (see Figure 3-8): Pleurovac components: 3 chambers (previously were bottles).

First chamber (nearest the patient) = Collection chamber—where whatever effluent from the pleural cavity is collected.

Second chamber (middle) = Water-seal chamber—allows air to bubble out from the pleural cavity but does not allow air into the chest. Bubbles in this chamber indicate air is in (or still entering) the pleural space.

Third chamber (attached to suction) = Suction regulator—height of water determines the amount of suction on the chest tube (when vacuum is applied to the chamber and there is bubbling in the water of the chamber).

Recurrence prevention: Pleurodesis decreases the recurrence rate significantly. You usually do pleurodesis with the first episode of SSP and typically reserve it for the second occurrence of PSP, but it is reasonable to use it for the first. There is more evidence suggesting that you should do pleurodesis for even the first occurrence of PSP, and this may become the standard of care. Talc is the best and cheapest means. Doxycycline and minocycline are next. Bleomycin is too toxic and no longer recommended.

SINUSITIS/TONSILLITIS

Acute sinusitis has the following usual causes: *S. pneumoniae*, *S. pyogenes*, and *H. influenzae*. The most common predisposing problem is a viral URI causing obstruction of the sinus outlets. Treat with TMP/SMX, AM/CL, clarithromycin, a 2nd/3rd generation cephalosporin, or fluoroquinolones. Treat recurrent sinusitis for 3 weeks. Osteomyelitis of the frontal bone is rare; it is indicated by a pale, cool edematous area over the forehead called Pott's puffy tumor.

Postanginal sepsis is an anaerobic sepsis secondary to thrombophlebitis of the jugular vein. This phlebitis is the result of spread from an adjacent tonsillar abscess.

PNEUMONIAS

OVERVIEW

Pneumonia is the most common infectious cause of death. Also see ARDS on pg 3-44.

First we will discuss the pneumonias categorized by pathogen, and then discuss assessment and treatment of nosocomial and the workup and empiric treatment of community-acquired pneumonias.

In this section on pneumonias, diagnosis and treatment will be highlighted in light BLUE and PINK, respectively.

BACTERIAL PNEUMONIAS: TYPICAL

Gram-Positive Pneumonias

Streptococcus pneumoniae

Streptococcus pneumoniae causes pneumococcal pneumonia. It comprises up to 50% of community-acquired pneumonias in the U.S. when a cause is identified. The patients typically present with a hard, shaking chill and pleuritic chest pain. Lab reveals a high WBC count (or very low WBC count if there is an overwhelming infection). Sputum may be rusty colored. Chest x-ray often shows lobar consolidation.

When is mortality increased in pneumococcal pneumonia? When the patient is elderly or alcoholic, when there is an underlying illness, when the infiltrate is multilobar, when the patient is bacteremic, or when the patient has WBCs < 5,000. If bacteremic, mortality is 30%! Despite antibiotics, this never has improved! In overwhelming pneumococcal sepsis, antibiotics do not make a difference as to whether the patient lives or dies in the first 24 hours!

The pneumococcal vaccine indications are discussed under Preventive Medicine in the General Internal Medicine section.

Gram stain is positive if there are lancet-shaped Gram-positive diplococci in a sputum sample that also have many PMNs and < 10 epi's per low-power field—best if organisms are intracellular. Do not be fooled by the slide with many epithelial cells; this is just spit, and non-diagnostic, no matter what else you may see on it (more on this later).

Drug-resistant *S. pneumoniae* is more likely with: age > 65 yrs, recent β-lactam therapy, alcoholism, immunosuppression, multiple comorbidities, and exposure to child in daycare.

Diagnosis of *S. pneumoniae* pneumonia may be confirmed with a sputum Gram stain and C+S. A positive blood culture is helpful. The pneumococcal urinary antigen assay (IDSA, 2003) may also be done and will augment the diagnosis.

30% of *S. pneumoniae* are at least somewhat resistant to β-lactams (including methicillin)! Even so, high-dose amoxicillin is considered adequate empiric coverage. This is because the original determinations of resistance to the β-lactams was done on levels achievable in the CSF (for meningitis), not the lung. [Levels for amoxicillin, ceftriaxone, and cefotaxime have been restated but not those for PCN, which has the same effectiveness—e.g., making amoxicillin look > 20x as effective as PCN...Yikes!]

Drug resistance in *S. pneumoniae* (DRSP) is becoming significant not only with β-lactams (as above), but also with fluoroquinolones, and macrolides.

Effective antibiotics for *S. pneumoniae* are the antipneumococcal fluoroquinolones (levofloxacin, gatifloxacin, moxifloxacin, and gemifloxacin), high-dose amoxicillin or PCN, and advanced macrolides (azithromycin and clarithromycin).

Staphylococcus aureus

Staphylococcus aureus is usually seen in patients with a preceding influenza infection or in patients who have been on antibiotics to which *S. aureus* is resistant. Patients typically present with a low WBC count and often are septic. The sputum may have blood in it and be "salmon pink." Chest x-ray shows patchy infiltrates and occasionally cavitation. Complications include empyema (frequent), an immune-complex type of glomerulonephritis, and pericarditis.

Diagnose *S. aureus* pneumonia with a sputum Gram stain and C+S. Also do blood cultures if suspected.

Treatments are: 1st generation cephalosporin or penicillinase-resistant, synthetic penicillin (nafcillin). Vancomycin if MRSA is suspected —until C&S is back.

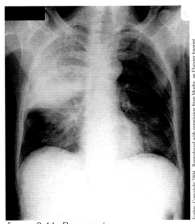

Forbes, Copyright 2004. Reproduced with permission from Mosby, an Elsevier Imprint

Image 3-11: Pneumonia

Gram-Negative Pneumonias

Enteric Gram-negative

Enteric Gram-negative—especially *Klebsiella*, *E. coli*, and *Proteus*. 30% of pneumonias in elderly patients (especially nursing home patients) are caused by enteric Gram-negative organisms. These pneumonias are often rapidly fatal, and patients often present in septic shock. Sputum may include a mixture of blood and pus, giving it the classic "currant jelly" appearance.

Chest x-ray: *Klebsiella* may show a bulging fissure sign. *Klebsiella*, *E. coli,* and *Proteus* usually do not cavitate.

Enteric Gram-negative (especially *Klebsiella*) pneumonia is associated with: nursing home resident, cardiopulmonary disease, recent antibiotic therapy, multiple comorbidities.

Diagnose enteric Gram-negative pneumonias with sputum Gram stain and C+S.

Treatment of enteric Gram negatives is based on C+S. Newer fluoroquinolone or, if sick, piperacillin + tazobactam is preferred therapy.

Pseudomonas aeruginosa

Pseudomonas aeruginosa is the most common infection acquired while on a mechanical ventilator. Even so, know that *Pseudomonas* often colonizes the airway of patients on ventilators, but this alone is no reason to treat these patients with antibiotics! Patient risk factors are steroid treatment, recent use of broad-spectrum antibiotics, CHF, and malnutrition.

Pseudomonas aeruginosa pneumonia is associated with: Bronchiectasis, corticosteroid therapy, broad-spectrum antibiotic therapy for > 7 days in past month, malnutrition, and recent hospitalization—especially in the ICU.

Diagnose *Pseudomonas aeruginosa* pneumonia with sputum Gram stain and C+S.

Treat with 2 synergistic antipseudomonal agents, such as an aminoglycoside + an antipseudomonal beta-lactam (i.e., gentamicin plus ceftazidime or cefoperazone or piperacillin or ticarcillin).

Haemophilus influenzae

Haemophilus influenzae may be encapsulated or unencapsulated. It is rarely seen in community-acquired pneumonias; usually you see it in the elderly—especially COPD patients. *H. influenzae* may cause recurrent infections in patients with immunoglobulin deficiency (especially IgG).

Diagnose *Haemophilus influenzae* pneumonia with sputum Gram stain and C+S. Sputum Gram stain shows Gram-negative coccobacilli.

Antibiotics effective against *H. influenzae* are ampicillin (or AM/CL if resistance is suspected or common in your area), 3rd generation cephalosporins, doxycycline, fluoroquinolones, and TMP/SMX.

Moraxella catarrhalis

Moraxella catarrhalis (formerly *Branhamella*, which was formerly *Neisseria*) is usually seen in patients with chronic bronchitis, COPD, DM, cancer, or in patients taking corticosteroids.

Diagnose *Moraxella catarrhalis* pneumonia with sputum Gram stain and C+S. Sputum Gram stain shows Gram-negative cocci.

Antibiotics: doxycycline, macrolide, cephalosporin, or AM/CL. Up to 90% of isolates produce a beta-lactamase, which breaks down penicillin but not cephalosporin.

ATYPICAL PNEUMONIAS

Overview

Atypical pneumonias usually occur in younger patients. Patients typically have no sputum production, a nontoxic appearance, and normal or slightly elevated WBCs. Atypical pneumonia may follow an upper respiratory infection. Atypical pneumonias can be caused by *Mycoplasma*, *Chlamydophilia pneumoniae* (TWAR), *Chlamydophilia psittaci* (bird farmers), *Legionella*, *Histoplasma*, *Coccidioides*, and viruses. Other causes include Q fever and tularemia. Think of

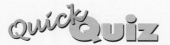

tularemia in patients who hunt or skin animals. Think of Q fever if the patient works around cattle or sheep; these animals are naturally infected, but the causative organism, *Coxiella burnetii*, is not transmitted between humans.

Mycoplasma pneumoniae

Mycoplasma pneumoniae is the cause of ~ 20% of community-acquired pneumonias in young patients. Having a 2–3 week incubation period, it spreads slowly (person-to-person). It usually has an insidious onset, with the chest x-ray often appearing worse than the symptoms suggest. Occasionally, it has a more acute onset and can mimic a pneumococcal pneumonia.

Extrapulmonary manifestations of *Mycoplasma* pneumonia include hemolytic anemia, splenomegaly, erythema multiforme (and Stevens-Johnson syndrome), arthritis, myringitis bullosa, pharyngitis, tonsillitis, and neurologic changes—especially confusion.

Diagnosis: Complement fixation—which mainly measures IgM antibody. Do not use cold agglutinins, which are neither sensitive nor specific.

Treatment of *Mycoplasma* pneumonia: macrolide—doxycycline if the macrolide is not tolerated. Patients sometimes take a long time (> 6 months) to fully recover!

Chlamydophilia pneumoniae

Chlamydophilia pneumoniae (formerly *Chlamydia*) causes epidemic pneumonia in young adults. It may be the cause of up to 10% of community-acquired pneumonias. Symptoms are similar to *Mycoplasma* pneumonia with the addition of laryngitis. Often, there is a biphasic illness; the patient presents with a sore throat that is negative for group A *Strep*; then 2–3 weeks later, pneumonia develops.

Diagnosis of pneumonia due to *Chlamydophilia pneumoniae* is confirmed with a single IgM titer > 1:16 using microim-

munofluorescence (MIF) test, positive culture, PCR of respiratory secretions, or a 4-fold increase in IgG titer. The first 3 are most useful clinically.

Effective antibiotics include doxycycline and macrolides for 3 weeks.

Legionella pneumophila

Legionella pneumophila causes up to 15% of CAPs. It is the cause of 1–5% of patients hospitalized for community-acquired pneumonia. It is picked up in cool damp places, such as near water coolers, and has a predilection for winter and summer months. It can even be carried on hospital shower heads! *Legionella pneumophila* causes legions of problems. Multisystem disease is the clue! Patients often have diarrhea and CNS symptoms (H/A, delirium, and confusion) presenting in addition to the pneumonia.

Presentation is similar to, and often confused with, *Mycoplasma pneumoniae*. Like *M. pneumoniae*, the CXR is much worse-looking than the exam indicates.

Think of this if the patient has fever, diarrhea, pneumonia, and headache or altered mental status. Or the patient has an "enigmatic" (mystifying) pneumonia. It is associated with low serum Na^+ and PO_4.

Preferred diagnostic tests for *Legionella pneumophila* pneumonia are sputum culture on special media and the urinary antigen assay. Urinary antigen assay has less sensitivity with milder disease.

Treatment: macrolides—especially azithromycin or quinolones. If severely ill, add rifampin as initial treatment.

Coccidioides immitis

Coccidioides immitis infection (coccidioidomycosis) is endemic in the Southwestern U.S. (C for California). The infection is also called "valley fever." Spores grow best in arid, desert-like climates ("valley fever" comes from association with the San Joaquin valley). Erythema nodosum and erythema multiforme commonly occur in infected people. A typical presentation is a person with erythema multiforme and a history of travel to the Southwest.

To even think of *Coccidioides*, you must get a good travel history—so do one in all patients with pneumonia! Diagnose by immunodiffusion (gel diffusion).

Treatment of coccidioidomycosis: the common, self-limited form usually does not require treatment and may leave thin-walled lung cavities. Treat with fluconazole and/or amphotericin B if there is hemoptysis or enlargement on chest x-ray.

Disseminated coccidioidomycosis is seen in immunocompromised/HIV. This is a fulminant disease with meningitis and with skin and bone involvement. Even with treatment (amphotericin B), it is frequently fatal.

Histoplasma capsulatum

Histoplasmosis is uncommon, except in endemic areas of the South and Midwestern U.S. It is especially seen in the Mississippi and Ohio River valleys (but do not confuse this with "[San Joaquin] valley fever" above). Think of "histoplas-

MOsis" (Mississippi, Ohio). It is associated with soil animals (chickens) and cave-dwelling animals (bats).

With acute disease, the chest x-ray shows hilar adenopathy and focal alveolar infiltrates. Heavy exposure ("epidemic," disseminating form) is suggested by a chest x-ray revealing multiple nodules in addition to the hilar adenopathy.

Diagnose histoplasmosis with:
1) If systemic disease, use antigen test of the blood, BAL, or urine.
2) If pneumonia, use serologic tests. Complement fixation is more sensitive than immunodiffusion.

No treatment is indicated for the usual disease, although some recommend itraconazole. Disseminating disease requires amphotericin B.

Blastomyces dermatitidis

Blastomycosis is uncommon. It is usually acquired by middle-aged men in the Central, Southeast, and Mid-Atlantic states (think of having a "blast" in Chicago). M:F is 10:1! Progression can be indolent to severe. Chest x-ray shows infiltrates that appear mass-like.

Diagnosis of blastomycosis: No skin test is available. Blastomycosis is more pyogenic than the others—patients can have purulent sputum—which reveals large, single-budding yeasts (KOH).

Treatment:
• Indolent: observe or oral itraconazole
• Mild-to-moderate: itraconazole x 6 months; also can use ketoconazole or fluconazole.
• Severe: amphotericin B; then may switch to itraconazole. HIV patients require chronic suppression with itraconazole

VIRAL PNEUMONIAS

Influenza

Viruses—Influenza A and B are still the most common viral causes of lung infection in adults. Age > 65 years is a big risk factor for increased mortality. Other viral causes of pneumonia include adenoviruses (also frequent) and CMV.

Influenza vaccination and prophylaxis is covered under Preventive Medicine in the General Internal Medicine section.

Diagnose influenza A and B with rapid antigen detection assay—especially recommended is an assay that distinguishes between influenza A and B.

Amantadine and rimantadine are now ineffective for influenza, and oseltamivir (Tamiflu®) and zanamivir (Relenza®) are recommended now for both A and B.

Influenza often leads to superinfection with a bacterium. If so, cover for S. pneumoniae, S. aureus, and H. influenzae.

Severe Acute Respiratory Syndrome

There was an outbreak of SARS between March and July 2003 in China, Hong Kong, Vietnam, Singapore, Thailand, and Canada (Toronto), but only sporadic cases since then.

Diagnosis of SARS: if indicated, do diagnostic studies for the coronavirus. These include sputum culture, acute IgM antibody, and SARS coronavirus RNA detection by PCR x 2.

Treatment: Supportive care. Some tests suggest that interferon-alpha plus corticosteroids are effective.

ASPIRATION SYNDROMES

With aspiration syndromes, infection usually occurs only after a large amount of material is aspirated—e.g., after endotracheal intubation, seizures, or in a severely intoxicated patient. The infiltrate usually occurs in the RLL. When a patient aspirates, it is not necessary to start antibiotics immediately, because stomach contents often cause only a chemical pneumonitis. Even so, observe the patient carefully, because cavitating pneumonia and/or empyema can develop. The breath can be horrendously malodorous in those with infection!

Gram smear shows mixed flora. Sputum is unreliable. Most common infection-causing bacteria are Fusobacterium nucleatum, Bacteroides melaninogenicus, and anaerobic Streptococcus.

Treatment: The antibiotic used for aspiration pneumonia must cover anaerobes, which usually are the cause of cavitation. Amoxicillin/clavulanate or clindamycin are generally recommended.

If an alcoholic patient with poor dentition presents with a severe cavitating pneumonia localized to the superior segment of the RLL, what is the cause?...Right! What is the treatment?...Right! ("Right," that is, if you said anaerobes and amoxicillin/clavulanate or clindamycin)

NOSOCOMIAL PNEUMONIAS

There are 3 types of "nosocomial" pneumonia:
1) Hospital-acquired (HAP) if it occurs 48 hours or more after admission.
2) Ventilator-associated pneumonia (VAP) is defined as occurring more than 48–72 hours after endotracheal intubation.
3) Healthcare-associated pneumonia (HCAP) occurs in a patient who was either hospitalized in an acute care hospital for 2 or more days within 90 days of developing the pneumonia; resided in a long-term care facility; received IV antibiotics, chemotherapy, or wound care within 30 days prior to the pneumonia; or attends a hospital or hemodialysis clinic.

Bacterial pneumonias are the most common types of nosocomial pneumonias, especially those due to enteric Gram-negative organisms. Elderly patients are more susceptible. Strep pneumoniae, Staph aureus, including MRSA (methicillin-resistant S. aureus), and H. influenzae are next most common; Strep pyogenes and the Klebsiella species are now uncommon.

notes

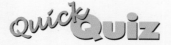

COMMUNITY-ACQUIRED PNEUMONIAS

Overview

There are about 4 million cases of community-acquired pneumonia (CAP) yearly and 25% are hospitalized. [Know all of this section very well!]

CAP is most often found to be due to *S. pneumoniae* (~ 50%), with the other causes being *Mycoplasma* and other atypical organisms, viruses, *S. aureus*, *H. influenzae*, enteric Gram-negative organisms, anaerobes, and other miscellaneous causes. Anaerobic causes are probably under-represented, because they are usually not included in routine screening tests. It is difficult to put a percentage on the causes, because they can vary widely depending on the time of the year, age of the patients, and region.

Diagnosis of CAP

Review of symptoms: Atypical pneumonias (~ 20% of CAPs) usually have an insidious onset with predominance of constitutional symptoms. The cough is usually non-productive, whereas bacterial pneumonias typically have an abrupt onset of symptoms; respiratory symptoms predominate, normally with a large amount of purulent sputum. There is such overlap in symptoms that you cannot use the history of symptoms to differentiate between atypical and bacterial pneumonias.

[Know]:

The chest x-ray is required for diagnosis of CAP; a new infiltrate along with new cough (+/- fever, etc.) indicates CAP. Some confusion in reading the chest x-ray may result from CHF, COPD, and malignancy. Also, an infiltrate may not appear in a volume-depleted patient.

Sputum tests: Do a sputum Gram stain and C+S, and an acid-fast stain if indicated. The C+S results are accurate only if there are < 10 epi's per low-power field (if > 25 epi's, do not even bother culturing—it is too contaminated!). Best results are obtained if the specimen also contains > 25 WBCs per low-power field. If the patient gives you a cup with what looks like saliva mixed with a few mucoid globs, fish out these "goobers" and send them to the lab (higher yield)!

Two pretreatment blood cultures should be done on admitted patients. Additional admission tests are: CBC, Chem-6, liver function tests, O_2 sat, and HIV testing (if 15–54 years old and you have consent).

Not done initially: Serologic tests are usually not helpful in the initial evaluation. DNA probes and nucleic acid amplification are not indicated.

Treatment of CAP

Overview

The Guidelines from the American Thoracic Society (ATS) and Infectious Disease Society of America (IDSA) are the most commonly used for treatment of CAP. The most recent ATS Guidelines are from 2001, while the most recent IDSA guideline update is from 2003. The next set of guidelines for CAP will be a joint project from these two organizations.

See the diagram on the next page for an adaptation of the ATS guidelines for CAP with the IDSA guidelines indicated by strikethroughs and brown text. The IDSA guidelines are very similar.

The best way to assess and treat CAP is by a successful C + S. Even so, empiric treatment is started before pathogen identification, and this is based on:
- severity of the illness and need for hospitalization, and
- likelihood of a certain pathogen based on modifying risk factors.

PSI

Severity of the pneumonia is determined by the PORT (patient outcome research team) pneumonia severity index (PSI) that ranges from I to V. It is a determination of outcomes based on initial presentation, and it is now routinely used to determine the severity of pneumonia and whether the patient needs to be admitted to the hospital.

This determination is a two-step process. The first step is to see if the patient is in risk category I; this is determined solely from the history and physical exam. Basically, if there is no history of comorbidity and the physical exam is okay (normal mental status, pulse < 125, RR < 30, systolic BP $\geq$ 90, and temp $\geq$ 35 but < 40°C), then the patient is risk category I.

If the patient is not assigned to risk category I, the next steps are to do blood tests (Na, Glu, BUN, Hct, ABG are used in the PSI) and note from the x-ray how many lobes are affected and if there is a pleural effusion. Based on these results, the patient is put in risk category II–V. See Table 3-7. Note the jump in mortality rate for risk category IV and V compared to I–III! For this reason, those with a risk category of IV or V are admitted. Those with I–III are treated as outpatients.

Figure 3-9: Treatment of Inpatient and Outpatient Community-Acquired Pneumonia

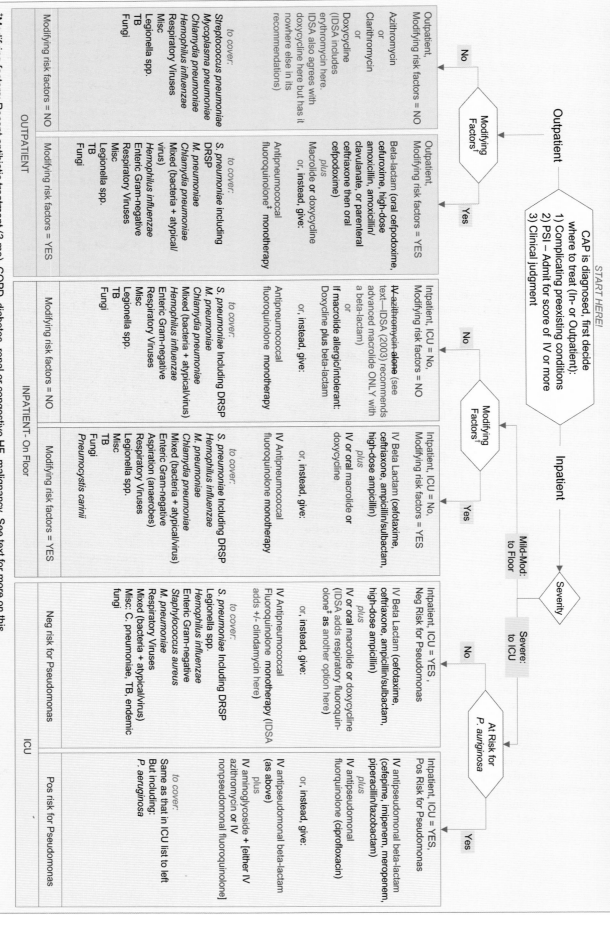

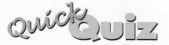

1) What are the risk factors for enteric Gram-negative CAP?

2) When is CAP due to *P. aeruginosa* more likely?

3) Know the usual choices for empiric therapy for patients with CAP—for outpatients and inpatients with and without the modifying factors that increase risk of DRSP or enteric Gram-negatives and for those in the ICU with and without increased risk for *P. aeruginosa* (Know this *and next page*).

First, we will review the modifying factors and then empiric therapy in order of increasing severity and risk factors, starting with the community-acquired pneumonias (CAP). Throughout this discussion on CAP follow along with the treatment flowchart shown in Figure 3-9. Read the footnotes to this flowchart before you start looking at it.

Table 3-7: The Pneumonia POST Severity Index

	Findings	Points Assigned
Demographic Factors	Males Females Nursing home residents	Age (in years) Age minus 10 Age +10
Comorbid Illnesses	Neoplastic disease Liver disease Congestive heart failure Cerebrovascular disease Renal disease	+ 30 + 20 + 10 + 10 + 10
Physical Exam	Altered mental status Resp rate $\geq$ 30 bpm Systolic BP < 90 mmHg Temp < 35°C or $\geq$ 40°C Pulse $\geq$ 125 bpm	+ 20 + 20 + 20 + 15 + 10
Laboratory	pH < 7.35 BUN > 10.7 mmol/L Na < 130 Glucose > 139 Hct < 30% PO$_2$art < 60 mmHg or O$_2$sat < 90% Pleural effusion	+ 30 + 20 + 20 + 10 + 10 + 10 + 10

Scoring	Points	Mortality (%)
I	< 51	< 0.5
II	51-70	$\geq$ 0.5, <1.0
III	71-90	$\geq$ 1.0, < 4.0
IV	91-130	$\geq$ 4.0, < 10.0
V	> 130	$\geq$ 10.0

Pathogens Associated With Modifying Factors

Drug-resistant *S. pneumoniae* (DRSP) pneumonia is more likely:
Age > 65 yrs, recent (3 mo) β-lactam therapy, alcoholism, immunosuppression, multiple comorbidities, and/or exposure to child in daycare.

Enteric Gram-negative (especially *Klebsiella*) pneumonia is more likely:
Nursing home resident, cardiopulmonary disease, recent antibiotic therapy, and/or multiple comorbidities.
Pseudomonas aeruginosa pneumonia is more likely in:
Bronchiectasis, corticosteroid therapy, broad-spectrum antibiotic therapy for > 7 days in past month, malnutrition, and recent hospitalization—especially in the ICU.

You must also take into account the patient's history, as well as the current landscape of pathogens and their antibiotic sensitivities at your hospital and in your community.

Other historical factors:
• COPD patient or the patient with immunoglobulin deficiency, especially IgG: consider *Moraxella catarrhalis* (formerly *Branhamella*) and *H. influenzae*.
• Cattle or sheep exposure: consider Q fever.
• Bird farmers: think of psittacosis.
• Hunters: consider tularemic pneumonia.
• Bat caves in the Mississippi and Ohio River valleys: histoplasMOsis.
• Travel to California or Arizona: Coccidioidomycosis.
• Chicago (central, southeast, and mid-Atlantic states): blastomycosis.
• Homosexual: PCP

Empiric Therapy

Overview

Empiric therapy is based on where the patient is being treated, the modifying factors that make certain pathogens more likely, and, when in the ICU, if *P. aeruginosa* is a risk. β-lactams are never given as monotherapy because they lack activity against the atypical pathogens. Antibiotic selection is the same for elderly patients with CAP as for all adults.

Macrolide resistance is now seen in 20–30% of *S. pneumoniae*, and it may even occur during therapy! There is also a concern for increasing resistance with the use of fluoroquinolones.
So again, know the specifics about the pathogens going around in your community, and take this knowledge into account when you start empiric therapy for CAP.
Treatment should be started within 4 hours of admission for inpatients.
Know empiric therapy of CAP well! The rest of this section is an explanation of the chart on the opposite page discussing empiric treatment of CAP. Refer to the diagram as we go through this information.

Outpatients

Basically, the majority of patients with CAP are treated as outpatients—usually with either macrolides (azithromycin or clarithromycin) or doxycycline.

Note that the IDSA includes erythromycin as a choice, but GI side effects limit its use, and it is less effective against *H. influenzae* than the advanced macrolides.

The IDSA agrees that doxycycline is an option for outpatients with no modifying risk factors, but does not include doxycycline as a recommendation in any other case—this is probably because, even though doxycycline does exhibit good activity against these pathogens, there are limited clinical trials of doxycycline for CAP (who will fund them now?…it's generic!) and these guidelines are evidence-based as much as possible. (Ah-Ha! the drug companies' plan is working!)

If they have risk factors, such as recent antibiotic therapy, DRSP is more of a concern and a specific β-lactam, effective against DRSP, is added. Alternately, monotherapy with an antipneumococcal fluoroquinolone is given.

Note: Even high-dose amoxicillin is a suitable empiric therapy if DRSP is suspected, because DRSP is usually only somewhat resistant to β-lactams.

Inpatients—non-ICU

Inpatients on the floor are all treated pretty similarly for CAP. Note that the azithromycin monotherapy recommendation has been dropped because of the increasing resistance of *P. pneumoniae* to macrolides, and because recent studies have shown significantly lower mortality if the macrolide is combined with a cephalosporin. Instead, the IDSA recommends advanced macrolides (azithromycin or clarithromycin) plus a β-lactam. All floor patients with CAP have the option of a respiratory fluoroquinolone monotherapy.

Note: If the inpatient came in from a nursing home, enteric Gram-negative organisms are a concern and treatment should consist of:
1) respiratory (antipneumococcal) fluoroquinolone monotherapy, or
2) high-dose amoxicillin-clavulanate plus an advanced macrolide (azithromycin or clarithromycin).

Inpatients—ICU

Empiric CAP treatment for the ICU patient (with no risk factors for pseudomonas) is about the same as that for the floor patient who has modifiers. The IDSA gives another couple of options:
1) β-lactam with a respiratory fluoroquinolone
2) Respiratory fluoroquinolone +/- clindamycin

If the ICU patient has risk factors for *P. aeruginosa*, the antibiotics must cover it.

LUNG ABSCESS

In general, lung abscesses have the same etiology as pneumonias. Only rarely are they caused by hematogenous spread.

Anaerobic pathogens are the most common cause of empyema and lung abscesses; the lung abscesses usually result from aspiration pneumonia. In IV drug abusers, septic pulmonary emboli often cause lung-abscess formation; these emboli are usually from a tricuspid valve infection but can also be from an infected injection site. Infected AV shunts are a cause of septic emboli in renal failure patients.

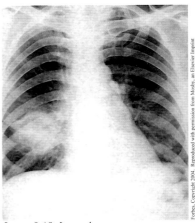

Image 3-12: Lung abscess

MYCOBACTERIAL INFECTION
TUBERCULOSIS

Overview

Much of the following on tuberculosis (TB) is adapted from the CDC/ATS Statement committee reports. You can download them from http://www.cdc.gov/mmwr.

TB is a favorite board topic. For good reason—the incidence of TB has been increasing since 1988. This is mainly due to TB associated with HIV infections.

The infection sequence goes: primary infection → latent infection → reactivation.

Tuberculosis infection occurs when aerosolized, contaminated droplets (coughed up by a diseased person) are inhaled by another and the droplet, or droplet nuclei, reaches an alveolus. This is almost always a latent infection called latent tuberculosis infection (LTBI). It may be an active infection in HIV patients. Know that we no longer do "prophylaxis" after a positive PPD but rather "treat" the LTBI.

"Reactivation" TB may occur days-to-years later, if at all. 90% remain disease-free. The risk of conversion is 5% within 2 years and another 5% thereafter. HIV patients are an exception and have 40% risk of conversion within several months.

Primary TB infection—commonly seen in HIV patients—is primarily a lower-lobe disease (reflecting the site of initial infection which is due to increased airflow to the lower lobes in normal lungs).

Latent TB infection (LTBI) has no physical findings.

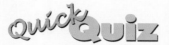

1) Define the differences between primary TB infection, LTBI, and reactivation TB.

2) What is miliary TB? What are the chest x-ray findings?

3) Give some examples of the group of people in whom a 5 mm PPD reaction is considered positive.

Reactivation tuberculosis is primarily an upper lobe and/or apical disease. See Image 3-13 and Image 3-14

Common presenting signs of reactivation tuberculosis include fever, weakness, night sweats, and weight loss. Pulmonary disease is indicated by cough, pleuritic chest pain, and hemoptysis. The chest x-ray may show an upper lobe infiltrate and hilar lymphadenopathy. Acid-fast stains of the sputum may show "red snappers;" you can also send sputum for PCR and culture. Most reactivation tuberculosis is pulmonary; 15% is extrapulmonary. Consider TB in a patient with chronic arthritis or meningitis refractory to treatment.

Report all persons with current reactivation tuberculosis or suspected current reactivation tuberculosis to the state or local health department.

Miliary tuberculosis is the term given to uncontrolled hematogenous spread of *M. tuberculosis*. The clinical picture is variable—from mild to overwhelming disease with multiple organ failure. Usually it presents as a chronic wasting disease. The classic chest x-ray is a faint and diffuse reticulonodular infiltrate (see Image 3-15).

Screening for Latent TB Infection (LTBI)

Who gets screened? High-risk groups including:
- HIV or high-risk for HIV
- close contacts of those with reactivation tuberculosis
- IV drug abusers
- low-income, medically underserved populations
- the homeless
- migrant workers
- residents of long-term care facilities (nursing homes and jails)

How are they screened? 2 methods:
1) The tuberculin skin test is the best and most widely used.
2) For people easily lost to follow-up, such as in some jails and homeless shelters, screen for actual disease (chest x-ray and sputum for AFB). (Summarized in Table 3-8)

Notes: Tuberculin skin tests are positive in most infected people. The tuberculin skin test is contraindicated only if there has been a necrotic skin reaction to previous tests. It may be given if the patient has had the BCG vaccine (used in some non-U.S. countries as a TB vaccine). Because most of these people were vaccinated as infants, the PPD will probably be valid and should be interpreted and acted on accordingly.

The standard Mantoux test is an intradermal injection of 0.1 ml (5 tuberculin units) of purified protein derivative (PPD) tuberculin in the forearm. The injection site is evaluated 48–72 hours after the injection. The reading is based on the diameter of the indurated/swollen area—not the red area—measured perpendicularly to the long axis of the forearm.

The current recommendations from the CDC as to what constitutes a positive reading (listed below) take into account the degree of clinical suspicion of LTBI. The following list shows how a particular diameter of induration may test positive in one group and negative in another. All of the following are considered positive skin tests:

5 mm is positive for those in the high-risk group. The high-risk group includes persons with:
- HIV or major cell-mediated dysfunction
- fibrotic changes on CXR consistent with prior TB
- close contact with a documented case
- patients with organ transplants and other immunosuppressed patients (receiving the equivalent of ≥ 15 mg/d of prednisone for 1 month or more)

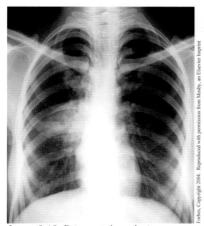

Image 3-13: Primary tuberculosis infection. Usually in the lower lobes.

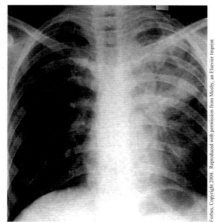

Image 3-14: Reactivation tuberculosis with LUL infiltrate

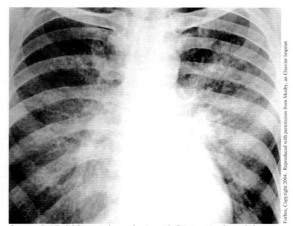

Image 3-15: Miliary tuberculosis with faint reticulonodular infiltrate

notes

10 mm is positive for those in the intermediate-risk group:
- homeless persons
- recent immigrants (within 5 years) from high prevalence countries
- IV drug abusers who are HIV-negative
- prisoners
- health care workers!
- nursing home patients and staff
- diabetics
- immunosuppressive therapy: equivalent to < 15 mg/d prednisone
- children < 4 years old

15 mm is positive for the low-risk group. This includes most people in the community.

Most concise way to remember this: HIV, + chest x-ray, close contacts, severely immunocompromised = 5 mm; no risk factors = 15 mm; all the rest = 10 mm.

False-negative skin tests. Think: A) too recent an exposure, or B) anergy.
A) It takes up to 10 weeks to turn positive after exposure so, if a recently exposed patient has a negative skin test, recheck 10–12 weeks after exposure. As discussed below, you treat this patient for LTBI until the second PPD is done and evaluated.

B) Previously, if anergy was suspected, 2 other skin tests (using antigens commonly reacted to) were done at the same time as the PPD. The validity of this has not proven out, and it is no longer recommended!

Booster Effect

Booster effect of TB skin tests: Some patients, especially the elderly who were infected with TB in the distant past, may no longer react to a TB skin test. Even so, the test may boost their immune system enough so that they react to subsequent skin tests. "2-step testing" has been devised to take advantage of this "booster" phenomenon.

Give elderly patients an initial test and, if negative, re-test in 1–3 weeks. If the second test is positive, assume they were infected with TB in the distant past and have active LTBI if not previously treated. If this negative patient has had recent exposure, recheck the skin test in 10–12 weeks, as you do with any other recently exposed negative reactor.

If the second test is negative, consider the patient to be free of established infection. It is a common practice to give the 2-step tuberculin test to all patients entering a nursing home for the first time.

Table 3-8: Positive PPD Determination based on Preexisting Conditions	
Treatment of Latent Tuberculosis Infection	
Certain groups are at high risk of developing TB *disease* once *infected*. These people are candidates for treatment *regardless* of their age -- after ensuring active infection is *not* present. The current optimum treatment regimen for *all* patients is 9 months of daily INH. See text for treatment of drug-resistant organisms. Treat ALL the following (ALL ages!):	
PPD Result (induration)	**In People with the Following Conditions**
≥ 5 mm is positive in this high-risk group	Known/suspected HIV infection Close contacts of active cases Chest radiograph suggests previous inactive tuberculosis Organ transplants and other immunosuppressed pts with greater than 1 month of equivalent prednisone use (> 15 mg/d)
≥ 10 mm is positive in these intermediate-risk groups	IV drug user known to be HIV-negative
	Immunosuppressive illness or therapy < 15 mg/d equivalent prednisone. Diabetes, Renal failure, or Hematologic malignancy.
	Immigrants from high-prevalence countries Residents of long-term care or correctional facilities Locally identified high-prevalence groups: migrant workers, homeless
≥ 15 mm is positive in this low-risk group	NO known risk factors
PPD negative but HIGH RISK	High risk contacts of ACTIVE cases

notes

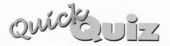

Quick Quiz

1) Give some examples of the group of people in whom a 10 mm PPD reaction is considered positive.

2) Give some examples of the group of people in whom a 15 mm PPD reaction is considered positive.

3) What do you do with a patient who was in close contact with a person with reactivation TB yet has a negative PPD?

4) Memorize Table 3-8!! This is important!!

5) What is the usual treatment (and for how long) for a 30-year-old patient with a positive PPD, a negative CXR and sputum, and a normal immune system?

6) How long should you treat with INH in a 30-year-old HIV-infected person with a positive PPD and negative CXR?

7) How long should you treat with INH in an 80-year-old man with a positive PPD and negative CXR?

8) Note that, in the above 3 questions, the patients are treated the SAME!

9) Again, how are close contacts of patients with active TB handled?

10) What is the treatment for most patients with reactivation TB?

Treatment of LTBI

Who Gets Treated for LTBI?

What do you do if the patient has a positive skin test? [Know!!] A positive skin test indicates that the patient has or has had LTBI, but not necessarily active disease. If the patient has had no previous TB workup, perform a workup for active disease: chest x-ray and a sputum for acid-fast bacteria (AFB) smear, PCR, and culture.

If the PPD is positive and active disease is present, treat for tuberculosis, as discussed in the next section.

If the PPD is positive and no active disease is present, treat all

previously untreated persons with the therapy options discussed below. This includes the 80-year-old and the 1-year-old. HIV-positive and HIV-negative. Recent or old seroconverters. (Simple, eh?)

How do you treat LTBI?

Treatment of LTBI: Give isoniazid (INH) to eradicate the TB infection before it can develop into the disease. Again, the risk of conversion is 5% within 2 years for normal persons and ~ 40% within several months for HIV patients. Optimal duration of treatment of LTBI is 9 months. See Table 3-8.

Treatment with INH is recommended for everyone except those with known exposure to INH-resistant organisms or history of INH intolerance. Instead, in these cases, give rifampin for 4 months. In the CDC's *Core Curriculum on TB* (2000), the recommendation is PZA + rifampin combination therapy—but this has proven too toxic and is no longer recommended (2002).

What about negative PPDs? Treat all persons with negative PPDs who are close contacts to patients with reactivation tuberculosis for 10–12 weeks, then recheck with another PPD. That's it!

Treatment of Reactivation Tuberculosis

Treatment: The emergence of multidrug-resistant strains has changed the treatment of reactivation tuberculosis. Let's first define the 4-drug and 3-drug regimens. [Know perfectly!]

The 4-drug regimen consists of:
• isoniazid (INH) • rifampin • pyrazinamide (PZA) and
• either ethambutol (oral—preferred) or streptomycin (injection)

The 3-drug regimen consists of the first 3 drugs (<u>I</u>NH, <u>Ri</u>fampin, and <u>P</u>ZA; <u>R</u>est <u>I</u>n <u>P</u>eace for the TB patient who doesn't get <u>R</u>ifampin, <u>I</u>NH, and <u>P</u>ZA).

In the U.S., all patients with reactivation tuberculosis are initially to be treated for 2 months with 4-drug therapy, unless criteria for 3-drug therapy are met (see below). Give the first 3 drugs for the full 2 months, while the 4th drug may be dropped if the susceptibility testing shows sensitivity to the first 3 drugs. After the first 2 months, give INH and rifampin for an additional 4 months. HIV-infected patients on protease inhibitors are usually given rifabutin instead of rifampin. Duration of therapy (6 months total) for HIV-infected patients is the same for those on a rifabutin regimen.

Give drugs daily for the first 2 months, then twice per week thereafter—although this is fairly flexible.

You must observe all patients taking the medication unless compliance is absolutely assured. The treatment is the same for extrapulmonary TB.

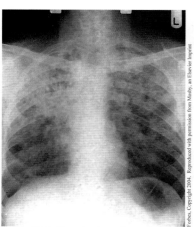

Image 3-16: Reactivation tuberculosis

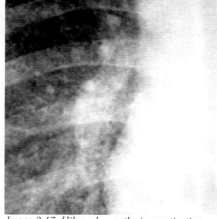

Image 3-17: Hilar adenopathy in reactivation tuberculosis

notes

When can 3 drugs be used? Only if there is a slight chance of drug-resistant infection. All the following criteria must be met:
- new TB patient and < 4% primary resistance to INH in the community
- no known exposure to a patient with a drug-resistant infection
- is not from a high-prevalence country

Also give Vitamin B$_6$ (pyridoxine) with INH-containing regimens to prevent peripheral neuropathy and mild central nervous system effects. Know the above recommendations cold; these are what's covered by the IM boards.

Some other scenarios:
- If the patient cannot take PZA, give INH and rifampin for a total of 9 months.
- If the TB is resistant to INH only, stop INH and give the other 3 drugs for 6 months (total) or rifampin and ethambutol for 12 months.
- Multidrug-resistant TB (i.e., to at least INH and rifampin) is difficult to treat. Treatment is based on sensitivities.

Side effects: INH, rifampin, and PZA are all hepatotoxic.
INH: In all patients on INH, regardless of age, monitor monthly only for signs and symptoms of liver toxicity. Laboratory testing is indicated only if signs or symptoms develop!

Ethambutol is not hepatotoxic, but it can cause a decrease in visual acuity. Often, decreased color perception is the first sign of this deterioration. It is usually reversible if the drug is quickly discontinued. Patients should have an ophthalmologic exam before treatment and periodic checks thereafter (Snellen chart, gross confrontation eye exam, and question the patient). Any inflammatory disease of the eyes is at least a relative contraindication for ethambutol.
Streptomycin is an older aminoglycoside. It tends to cause ototoxicity and nephrotoxicity.

NON-TB MYCOBACTERIAL DISEASES (NTM)

Mycobacterium kansasii

Mycobacterium kansasii affects immunocompetent persons, especially smokers and those with DM or silicosis. These are harder to treat—3 drugs (INH/RIF/ethambutol) are needed for 18 months.

M. avium complex

M. avium-intracellulare (MAI—also called MAC for *M. avium complex*) is an increasingly common cause of a distinct subtype of indolent infection in 50–80-year-old women with chronic cough but no underlying illness (normal immune status and no previous lung disease). CT shows a characteristic "tree-in-bud" pattern.
The preferred treatment for disseminated MAC is combination therapy with clarithromycin *plus* ethambutol *plus* rifabutin.
Gastrectomy patients and AIDS patients typically do poorly. Older women with the subtype of infection just mentioned

improve with treatment. There is no sure cure for any of these patients!

IMMUNOSUPPRESSED PATIENTS

IMMUNE DYSFUNCTION

Note: The following is covered in more depth in the Infectious Disease section.
Bacterial pneumonia is the most frequent cause of death in immunodeficient patients. Mortality is 50%.

Humoral dysfunction: B cell dysfunction or decreased antibodies are seen in most patients with ALL, CLL, and multiple myeloma. These patients are especially susceptible to encapsulated organisms, including *Strep pneumoniae, H. influenzae,* and meningococci.
Patients with hypogammaglobulinemia, asplenia, sickle cell, or abnormal complement also have a tendency to acquire infections caused by the encapsulated organisms (*H. influenzae, Strep pneumoniae,* and meningococci).

Cell-mediated dysfunction: T cell defects are seen in patients with AIDS, lymphoma, uremia, post-organ transplant, and after use of steroids or alkylating agents. These patients are susceptible to infections caused by *P. jiroveci* (PCP—previously *P. carinii*), *Mycobacteria,* viruses such as CMV and HSV, fungus (*Cryptococcus*), *Legionella,* and *Nocardia.* A minority of patients with ALL is of the T cell variant, and these may have a T cell deficiency.
You see decreased PMNs or neutrophil dysfunction in patients with AML, CML (the myelogenous leukemias), bone marrow transplant, and in others getting ablative chemotherapy. These patients tend to get infections of Gram-negative organisms: *Staphylococcus aureus, S. epidermidis, Corynebacterium jeikeium* (JK), and fungi (*Candida* and *Aspergillus*).

ORGAN TRANSPLANT

Organ transplant patients get the same infections as patients with T cell defects.
- During the first 30 days, patients most commonly get the usual nosocomial infections—especially Gram-negative pneumonias and *Legionella.*
- 1–4 months, *P. jiroveci* (previously *P. carinii*), CMV, and *Mycobacteria* infections appear.
- After 4 months, think of *P. jiroveci,* encapsulated organisms, fungus (*Aspergillus* and *Candida*), and viral infections (include herpes). Also, community-acquired infections are common.

CMV infection is usually donor-to-recipient. The majority of renal and cardiac patients get CMV infections. It is the most common cause of fever after transplant! It usually occurs 6–8 weeks after transplant. CMV typically causes only a mild infection, but it is also responsible for 20% of deaths in cardiac transplants! Diagnosis: Think of CMV if there is a mixed bag of "-itises," because patients often get concurrent pneumoni-

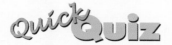

tis, hepatitis (usually mild), and adrenalitis-causing adrenal insufficiency! Finding inclusion bodies on BAL suggests the diagnosis. Finding inclusion bodies on a tissue sample (lung biopsy) confirms the diagnosis. Ganciclovir, along with high-dose IV immunoglobulin infusion, has been beneficial in bone marrow transplant patients.

MYELOPROLIFERATIVE DISORDERS

With regard to myeloproliferative disorders, if there is a localized infiltrate, it is usually caused by a bacterial pneumonia. This pneumonia is usually Gram-negative! Treat empirically.

PATHOGENS IN THE IMMUNOSUPPRESSED

The highest-to-lowest order of frequency of pulmonary infections in AIDS patients:

PCP > TB/MAI > Bacteria > CMV/HSV > Fungal

(Note: This is for AIDS patients, not HIV-infected only! For them, it is Bacteria/Tuberculosis first!)

With patients on highly active antiretroviral therapy (HAART), the order changes, and the most likely cause is the same as for other people—community-acquired pneumonia (CAP).

Pneumocystis jiroveci pneumonia (PCP—formerly *P. carinii*) is still the most common opportunistic infection in AIDS patients, although its incidence is declining due to better prophylactic and antiretroviral treatments. A history of PCP and/or a CD4 count of < 200 (or 14%) indicate greatest risk for PCP. Chest x-ray usually shows diffuse, bilateral, symmetrical interstitial + alveolar infiltrates. You can try CO diffusing capacity (DLCO) and gallium scan, but these are not used much.

Diagnosis: In AIDS patients, sputum examination with immunofluorescent monoclonal antibodies reveals the organism in 80% of cases, while BAL or transbronchial biopsy gets the rest. Other ways to examine sputum are Giemsa stain and Gomori methenamine silver stain.

Treatment: IV or oral TMP/SMX or IV pentamidine are effective! Try TMP/SMX first, because it can eventually be given orally. Another alternative is atovaquone. A majority of PCP patients improve on the initial course of therapy (usually 3 weeks), but a good number have intolerable side effects from either medication.

Corticosteroids given concomitantly with initiating anti-PCP treatment reduce the likelihood of respiratory failure and death in patients with moderate-to-severe pneumonia. Give steroids to PCP patients with a P_aO_2 < 70 or an A-a gradient > 35 !

Tuberculosis: The treatment is the same as for any other patient with TB (see pg 3-41). Most AIDS patients with TB come from areas where there is already a high prevalence of TB! TB is usually very effectively treated in AIDS patients! The most effective treatment for *M. avium-intracellulare* is to get the CD4 count > 100 (with anti-retroviral therapy) and initiate combination therapy against the MAI—usually using clarithromycin or azithromycin with rifabutin and ethambutol.

Aspergillosis (this is not ABPA, which is discussed on pg 3-20) is seen in patients with AML, ALL, Hodgkin disease, heart or bone marrow transplant, those chronically on corticosteroids, and those with granulocytopenia lasting > 25 days (slow growing!). Sputum is worthless because *Aspergillus* is often found in normal sputum. Nasal cultures are okay (pretty good sensitivity/specificity), but a lung biopsy is often necessary. Aspergillus invades the pulmonary blood vessels, causing a pulmonary infarct picture. It also tends to disseminate. Aspergillosis can cause pulmonary hemorrhage and, when it does, there is 80% mortality, so early diagnosis and treatment are mandatory. Again note: If the patient has been granulocytopenic (< 500) for > 25 days, think of aspergillosis.

Cryptococcosis is associated with Hodgkin disease, corticosteroids, and transplants, but not with PMN defects or neutropenia. Chest x-ray may show nodules or mass lesions.

C. neoformans in sputum means infection (contrary to *Aspergillus*). Needle aspiration and lung biopsy are also accurate means of diagnosing cryptococcal pneumonia. If found, perform a lumbar puncture to evaluate for CNS infection.

Coccidioides immitis is endemic in the Southwestern U.S. (C for California). These infections are common in patients with myeloproliferative disorders, Hodgkin disease, transplants, and AIDS.

Histoplasmosis is uncommon in AIDS patients unless they are from endemic areas, such as the Southern and Midwestern U.S. It is especially found in the Mississippi and Ohio River valleys.

Nocardia asteroides infections are usually seen in T cell deficient patients (not those with humoral deficiency) and in patients with alveolar proteinosis. The pulmonary lesions may cavitate. Brain abscesses and subcutaneous dissemination may occur. Treat with sulfonamides.

Candida pneumonia is very difficult to diagnose in immunosuppressed patients. *Candida* in the sputum is nonspecific. Very rare occurrence.

Pulmonary mucormycosis—patients with leukemia are at especially high risk. It is also seen in diabetics. This infection has a poor prognosis.

Reactivation infections:
Besides reactivation TB, toxoplasmosis, herpes infections, cryptococcosis, and strongyloidiasis can reactivate in the immunosuppressed.

NONINFECTIOUS INFILTRATES

Drugs may have cytotoxic or non-cytotoxic lung effects. Only cytotoxic reactions can cause an atypia of Type II alveolar cells.

Methotrexate is the most common cause of non-cytotoxic lung reactions and causes a hypersensitivity interstitial pneumonitis. Bleomycin is the most common cause of cytotoxic pulmonary toxicity. Gold-induced lung disease is reversible—just stop the drug. Bleomycin, amiodarone, and the nitrosoureas all cause dose-related pulmonary disease, while almost all other offending drugs have a hypersensitivity or idiosyncratic effect. Uremia, supplemental O_2, and radiation therapy exacerbate bleomycin lung toxicity. Transbronchial lung biopsy is the diagnostic procedure of choice, but it is usually not needed.

Crack cocaine can cause a hypersensitivity pneumonitis, diffuse alveolar hemorrhage, and bronchiolitis obliterans.

Hemorrhage is common in patients with AML—it can be the only cause of pulmonary infiltrates. But remember: In AML, rule out *Aspergillus* infection as the cause of the hemorrhage. (Also remember, hemorrhage may be caused by idiopathic pulmonary hemosiderosis, Goodpasture, SLE, and post-bone marrow transplantation.)

Leukemic pulmonary infiltrates most commonly occur in ALL, and they always imply a high percentage of blasts. Leukostatic infiltrates (globs of WBCs in the pulmonary vessels) occur in myeloid leukemias when the WBC count is > 100,000. 1/2 of lymphoma patients have infiltrates.

Radiation reactions in the lung usually present within 6 months of treatment; radiation pneumonitis occurs within 6 weeks.

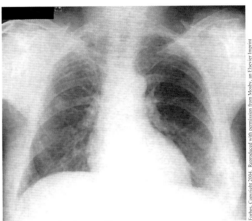

Image 3-18: Radiation fibrosis

CRITICAL CARE

ACUTE RESPIRATORY DISTRESS SYNDROME (ARDS)

Overview

Acute lung injury is defined as:
1) ratio of $P_aO_2/F_iO_2 \leq 300$, regardless of amount of PEEP
2) bilateral pulmonary infiltrates
3) PCWP ≤ 18 mg Hg (or no clinical evidence of left heart failure)

ARDS is defined as an acute lung injury in which the $P_aO_2/F_iO_2 \leq 200$. ARDS can have a direct or indirect precipitating event. Direct causes include aspiration, pneumonia, and inhalation injuries. Indirect events are sepsis, pancreatitis, multiple transfusions, and trauma. Aspiration and sepsis are the most common. With multiple precipitating events, risks increase.

A mnemonic:
• A (acute onset)
• R (restrictive lung mechanics)
• D (diffuse panendothelial inflammatory injury manifested in the lungs)
• S (shunt hypoxemia)

notes

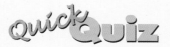
There is a 48–72 hour lag time between injury and ARDS. As yet, it is unknown what factors cause the leaky lungs in ARDS. In the septic patient with ARDS, it is thought that the endotoxin from the Gram-negative cell membrane activates complement, which in turn causes systemic endothelial damage. Tumor Necrosis Factor (TNF) and Interleukin-1 are monocyte-released mediators that probably help maintain the inflammatory state.

As yet, there is no prophylactic treatment for ARDS.

Death rate is 35–50% and decreasing. Death due to respiratory failure in ARDS is uncommon! The most common cause of death within the first 3 days after onset of ARDS is the underlying problem. After 3 days, sepsis is the most common cause of death—usually by way of multiple organ dysfunction/failure [Know!].

Making the diagnosis of pneumonia in the patient with ARDS is difficult, because infiltrates and leukocytosis are common in ARDS. Lavage fluid in ARDS without pneumonia has nearly 80% PMNs (normal < 5%). Growing $> 10^3$ organisms/ml in protected brush samples or $\geq 10^4$ organisms/ml in BAL samples is currently the best way to diagnose pneumonia in these patients. Give antibiotic therapy as indicated by BAL Gram stain and C + S results.

Prevention of pneumonia in the ARDS patient is important. Adequate handwashing and using sterile technique are mandatory. Antibiotic pastes and oral solutions do not appear to be effective.

Patients with ARDS tend to take 2 courses. They either get well quickly or their disease continues on to fibrotic lung injury.

Failure to improve pulmonary function in the 1st week is a negative prognostic sign.

Treatment

Treatment of ARDS: Treat the causative condition and provide optimized cardiopulmonary support. If the patient has an abscess, push surgeons to remove it or do interventional radiology to drain it. Give empiric antibiotics if sepsis is thought to be the cause. Keep patients slightly hypovolemic, but it is very important to provide enough volume to maintain adequate cardiac output and tissue-oxygen delivery—thereby preventing worsening lactic acidosis (and the resultant multi-organ failure). The optimum fluid management is currently undergoing trials.

Nutrition should be enteral rather than parenteral, if possible. There is not only less chance of catheter-induced sepsis, but enteral nutrition possibly prevents translocation of endotoxin and Gram-negative colonic bacteria.

Ventilator support for ARDS:

PEEP stands for positive end-expiratory pressure; on the ventilator, a valve shuts when the patient is near end-expiration, while there is still positive intrathoracic pressure.

The trouble with ARDS is that it has shunt physiology, and the only way to improve oxygenation is to recruit, or "pop open," some of the fluid-filled alveoli. At the same time, you want to avoid barotrauma and oxygen toxicity. To avoid oxygen toxicity, get $F_iO_2 < 60\%$ ASAP. To "pop open" alveolar units, use PEEP; but to avoid ventilator-induced lung injury (VILI), use adequate, but not excessive, PEEP.

Ventilator management has now changed with the recognition of the potential for ventilator-induced lung injury (VILI), which arises from overdistended alveoli (from a $\uparrow V_t$ or $\uparrow$ end-insp plateau press) and cyclic opening and closing of atelectatic alveoli (recruitment-derecruitment). Adequate level of PEEP prevents repetitive closure and opening of lung units. New recommendations from the NIH ARDS network (NEJM May 2000) indicate improved outcome with low tidal volumes (V_t) = 6 ml/kg and PEEP at adequate levels (discussed below). It turns out that maintaining low V_t appears to be critically important and, for now, 6 ml/kg is considered the optimal V_t. Generally, we start worrying about VILI due to excessive PEEP pressures at > 20–25 cm H_2O.

Previously, V_t in the range of 12–15 ml/kg had been used, but this is too high for many patients with ARDS, because their total lung capacity is much smaller than normal. There is a trend to lower tidal volumes in all patients on ventilators, whatever the cause.

No one ventilator has proven better than another for ARDS patients. An assist-control, volume-cycled ventilator is commonly recommended. Initial settings:

• F_iO_2 = 1 (then lower to < 60% ASAP)
• tidal volume (V_t) = start at 8 ml/kg ideal body weight and work down (6 is optimal). Monitor end-inspiratory plateau pressure!
• inspiratory flow = 60 L/min
• PEEP: a dose just greater than the lower inflection point on the ventilator PV curve. Some use an empiric regimen, in which they adjust the PEEP to maintain adequate S_aO_2 (arterial O_2 saturation) of at least 90% and low enough F_iO_2 (< 60%). PEEP usually starts at ≤ 5 cm H_2O, and usually goes up to 10–20 cm H_2O.

Positioning of the patient may help, especially if the infiltrate is not uniformly distributed. The lateral decubitus position is usually the first position tried. The prone position is problematic on a ventilator (!) but also may help. Data support increasing the P_aO_2/F_iO_2 ratio with prone positioning, which stabilizes the anterior chest wall causing improved physiology and recruitment of previously unused alveolar units. But there is no data yet to support decreased mortality.

Inverse ratio ventilation, in which inspiratory time is prolonged, may be useful in patients not responding to more conven-

notes

tional approaches. PEEP is very useful. See the following pages for more on ventilators, PEEP, and inverse ratio ventilation.

Permissive hypercapnia: The "ARDS Network low V_T protocol" is based on studies of (and is meant for) patients with acute lung injury (ALI) or ARDS. These study results show a 22% decrease in mortality!

The technique: Low V_T (tidal ventilation) with low V_E (expiratory flow) results in an elevated P_aCO_2 (permissive hypercapnia). The goal is to not worry about the P_aCO_2 so much as maintain adequate tissue oxygenation in an ARDS patient— maintain the $S_aO_2 > 88\%$. Although it is not necessarily related to PEEP, permissive hypercapnia is often started on ARDS patients requiring PEEP > 20 cm H_2O on conventional therapy. Hypercapnia is allowed to develop as needed to keep the PEEP no higher than 25 cm H_2O. Renal compensation for the respiratory acidosis usually ensues, and typically you do not need to give an alkali or increase the V_E. Permissive hypercapnia is used in severe exacerbation of obstructive lung disease as well. Again, the therapy-determining measurement is S_aO_2, not P_aCO_2.

Permissive hypercapnia is not used with intracranial hypertension or hemodynamic instability.

Nitric oxide at 5–80 ppm is a selective vasodilator and maintains vascular tone. 2 good studies show increase in P_aO_2/F_iO_2, but no survival benefit. It is currently not recommended.

Trials show no proven survival advantage in the following treatments for ARDS: high frequency ventilation, extracorporeal respiratory support, surfactant administration, NSAIDs, antiendotoxin therapy, and n-acetylcysteine (as an antioxidant).

To review ventilator use with ARDS, avoid:
• VILI
• oxygen toxicity

So first start V_t at 6 ml/kg, start F_iO_2 at 1 and reduce to < 60% ASAP. Use adequate but not excessive use of PEEP. Use permissive hypercapnia if needed.

Medications for ARDS:

Glucocorticoids have shown no benefit as a prophylactic before the onset of disease, nor in the early stages of ARDS. Glucocorticoids have shown some benefit as a treatment for the late fibroproliferative phase of the disease and for ARDS due to PCP (*P. jiroveci* [formerly *P. carinii*] pneumonia). Trials are ongoing. Even so, it is considered reasonable to use a short course of glucocorticoids as rescue therapy in severe cases that are not improving. They are sometimes tried with fat emboli-induced ARDS (controversial). Ensure there are no untreated infections.

Ketoconazole is a potent thromboxane inhibitor undergoing trials. It appears that it may be an effective prophylactic agent in patients at risk for ARDS. It does not affect outcome once the disease is present. No studies have been done to confirm the earlier promising studies of prophylaxis.

SEPSIS

Critically ill patients (especially sepsis +/- ARDS) can have a normal P_aO_2 and still have abnormal O_2 uptake by the tissues. This is thought to be a major contributor to multi-organ failure.

Hypophosphatemia decreases diaphragmatic contractility in addition to shifting the O_2 saturation curve to the left. Sucralfate can cause this!

Careful! Mixed venous O_2 may be misleading in the septic patient, because there is significant peripheral shunting. Lactic acid levels may be misleading as an indicator of tissue hypoxia, because an increase can also be caused by failure of the liver to clear it.

Always correct the underlying problem. You may do surgery/drainage on a focal infection if that is causing the sepsis, even if the patient is unstable.

Pulmonary artery catheterization utility is controversial in most cases of sepsis. PAWP reflects LVEDP, which affects stroke volume. Always read the PAWP at end-exhalation in these patients. Note: Read wedge pressure in all patients on a graphed wave form (not digital printout). Never take off PEEP to read the PCWP. More on PAWP in the Cardiology section.

MECHANICAL VENTILATION

Overview

The pressure in the cuff of the tracheal tube should be at the lowest possible pressure, ~15 mm Hg. When the pressure exceeds ~ 25 mm Hg, serious damage can occur to the tracheal mucosa.

Do a tracheostomy only after 2–3 weeks of intubation (barring other indications). Tracheostomy is not indicated to decrease airway resistance during weaning.

Ventilator-associated pneumonia is a frequent complication of mechanical ventilation. All patients are colonized with Gram-negative bacteria in upper and lower airways within 74–96 hours. It may be very difficult to sort out true pneumonia vs. colonization. For a diagnosis of pneumonia, you should see:
• new or increasing infiltrate,
• elevated WBCs,
• purulent sputum, and
• fever or hypothermia

Even with this clinical scenario, there is an ongoing debate about whether more invasive tests should be done to confirm the diagnosis. More invasive tests include PSB/BAL with quantitative cultures (PSB=Pulmonary double-sheathed brush). Antibiotic treatment must cover *Pseudomonas* in patients intubated ≥ 4 days.

Mechanical ventilation can be continuous or intermittent.

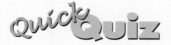

1) What is "permissive hypercapnia," and when is it used?

2) True or False: Tracheostomy is indicated to help reduce airway resistance in weaning.

3) Discuss the different modes of mechanical ventilation.

4) Name the "DESAT" causes of failure to wean.

5) A patient is failing to wean from the ventilator; you discover that she is on sucralfate. What laboratory value should you check?

Modes of Mechanical Ventilation

Continuous Mechanical Ventilation (CMV)

Controlled Ventilation has a set rate and set tidal volume that does not allow spontaneous breathing by the patient. Patient-ventilator asynchrony is a big problem and, therefore, this mode is best used for those patients who are under anesthesia, paralyzed with muscle relaxants, or in deep coma.

Assist/Control: This is a CMV with a set rate and tidal volume, but this mode allows the patient to initiate additional breaths. When the machine senses that the patient is attempting to take a breath, it will kick in with a full "machine breath" at the tidal volume you selected. This is a very commonly used mode of ventilation. One caveat is that, if patients are anxious and hyperventilating, they will continue to trigger additional full machine breaths, get even more hyperventilatory, and are at risk for developing auto-PEEP.

Intermittent Ventilation

SIMV: Synchronized Intermittent Mandatory Ventilation is similar to assist/control in that you dial in a set rate and tidal volume. If a patient takes a spontaneous breath, however, she does not get a machine breath; she gets only what she can generate on her own. Because this spontaneous breath asks a lot of work from your patient to suck in a breath through the endotracheal tube and the ventilator circuit, we often add "Pressure Support Ventilation (PSV)" to the SIMV mode so that, when the patient takes a spontaneous breath, she receives a boost of pressure (you set the amount) to help her overcome the resistance of the ETT and the ventilator circuit. Typically, use pressure support of 8–20 cm H_2O, but you need to titrate this pressure for an individual patient after you see what kind of spontaneous tidal volume the patient can generate.

Note: The above volume-cycled ventilators have a "pop-off" valve set at a certain inflation pressure to prevent over-pressurization of the lungs.

• PSV: Pressure Support Ventilation, as discussed above. In a spontaneously breathing patient, you can supply only pressure support, and there is no need for mandatory breaths.

This is a very comfortable mode for the patient in that he determines his respiratory rate and tidal volume. However, you must have a patient with a stable respiratory drive (i.e., not sedated heavily) and, most importantly, remember: There is no guarantee to the tidal volume that will be generated at a specific level of pressure support. If your patient is prone to—and develops—acute CHF, the lungs may acutely become "stiffer," and the unchanged level of pressure support will produce a much smaller tidal volume causing tachypnea and respiratory distress.

• Pressure Control: A newer form of ventilation that is actually a throwback to the first ventilators. Machine breaths are pressure-cycled, not volume-cycled. You determine the pressure you want the patient to receive on each breath and the rate at which the breaths will be delivered. If patient attempts a spontaneous breath, he will get a machine breath at the pressure you have designated. This may be helpful in limiting airway pressures in patients with high end-inspiratory plateau pressure in other volume-cycled modes that leave them susceptible to barotrauma. As with pressure support, there is no guarantee to the tidal volume and, hence, this mode must be titrated carefully at the bedside to determine the proper pressure settings.

Weaning and Failure to Wean

Weaning is now felt to be best accomplished using protocols. Generally, you do it in one of the following ways:

• SBT (Spontaneous Breathing with a T-tube) protocols generally recommend progressively longer periods of breathing on a T-tube—from 10 minutes to 2 hours. Usually, once the patient tolerates 2 hours on the T-tube, the ET tube is removed. SBT can also be accomplished on the ventilator (to allow tracking of RR, V_T, and V_E) using low level of PS (PS + 5 cm H_2O) or tube compensation.

• PSV (Pressure Support Ventilation), wherein the pressure is gradually reduced to the point where it is just overcoming the resistance of the ET tube. This is, in practice, pretty difficult to determine, because the resistance can vary from 3–14 cm H_2O (!) due to differing diameters and lengths, and kinks and deformations of the ET tube.

Failure to wean—possible causes (DESAT):
1) Drugs (sedatives...)
2) Endotracheal tube has too small a bore
3) Secretions
4) Alkalemia (decreases respiratory drive)
5) Too high a P_aO_2 and too low a PCO_2 just before extubating (should keep it near the patient's baseline).

Also consider diaphragm dysfunction caused by hypophosphatemia (e.g., from sucralfate), and the possibility of CHF. Stopping positive pressure ventilation → increased venous return → increased blood flow → increased cardiac output → CHF/cardiac ischemia in susceptible patients. COPD patients with respiratory failure are less able to get rid of CO_2, and CO_2 production is increased with fever and with large amounts of glucose and other carbohydrates in the diet. Se-

notes

vere COPD patients, then, may be harder to wean if they have a fever or have had a high carbohydrate diet.

Adjusting a Ventilator

Remember: When we are adjusting a ventilator to improve a patient's ABGs, we have to separate our actions into 2 categories [KNOW!]
- Those that change the Minute Ventilation (Respiratory Rate x Tidal Volume) = will change the patients pCO_2 and pH. Remember: Increased minute ventilation = decreased pCO_2
- Those that alter a patient's oxygenation: F_iO_2, PEEP, Inspiratory/Expiratory Ratio

PEEP

PEEP (Positive End-Expiratory Pressure) is a positive pressure left in the chest at the end of exhalation. This can be done purposely to a patient on a ventilator by closing a valve during exhalation, and not allowing the pressure in the airways to return to zero. You dial in a PEEP pressure—the desired end-expiratory pressure—typically 5–15 cm H_2O (can go higher in ARDS). The purpose of utilizing PEEP in mechanically ventilated patients is to help prevent the alveoli from completely collapsing at end-expiration. This prevents atelectasis and, more importantly, leads to better matching of V/Q while having less shunt fraction.

Use PEEP only with diffuse lung disease! It can actually decrease the P_aO_2 if used in focal lung disease. Use PEEP in cases of diffuse lung disease if required to maintain the F_iO_2 < 50%, while keeping the P_aO_2 > 60.

Too high a PEEP can cause:
- pneumothorax, ventricular failure, and alveolar damage, thereby precipitating or worsening pulmonary edema. The PEEP level recommended is just past lower inflection point on the pressure-volume curve;
- decreased venous return, causing decreased cardiac output and hypotension.

Auto-PEEP

Auto-PEEP usually happens when the time constant of the lung is violated in patients with high compliance and/or high airway resistance (high respiratory rate, high V_t, high bronchospasm).

In essence, the patients are not fully emptying their lungs during expiration prior to the initiation of the next breath. This is known as "stacking breaths" or generating auto-PEEP. A patient on a ventilator gets auto-PEEP if the ventilator is set up in a way so as not to allow the patient to fully exhale before initiating the next breath. This is particularly worrisome in patients who have exacerbations of COPD or status asthmaticus requiring mechanical ventilation. In ventilated patients, the auto-PEEP may become severe enough that the patient may suffer barotrauma or hemodynamic collapse due to the inability of blood to return to the chest. Auto-PEEP can be measured in mechanically ventilated patients:
- by inserting an end-expiratory pause in the ventilator circuit and observing the airway pressure monitor during the pause, or

- by using newer generation ventilators that automatically measure this for you at the touch of a button.

Treatment of auto-PEEP includes one or more of the following:
- decreasing respiratory rate
- decreasing V_t
- increasing TE (expiratory time)
- increasing PIFR (peak inspiratory flow rate)
- decreasing secretions

What do you do if your patient with severe airway obstruction has hypotension after being placed on mechanical ventilation?
1) Disconnect the patient from the ventilator and slowly bag the patient through the endotracheal tube. Check for tension pneumothorax, mucous plugs, and that the ventilator is functioning properly.
2) Return the patient to the ventilator with new settings that allow for a longer expiratory phase. Specific changes: lower the respiratory rate, increase the peak flow (shortening the time the patient gets for inspiration and, hence, allowing longer time for expiration), and reducing the tidal volume being delivered.

Note that the patient must be sedated or sedated + paralyzed to adequately measure auto-PEEP.

Inverse Ratio Ventilation

In ARDS, it has been proposed that we purposely generate auto-PEEP in patients with refractory hypoxemia as a means for splinting open or "recruiting" alveoli. This mode of ventilation is called inverse ratio ventilation and involves manipulating the I/E ratio (Inspiratory/Expiratory ratio) from the traditional 1:3, to ratios of 1:1, or even "flipped" ratios of 2:1 or 3:1. This can be done in either a volume-cycled (assist-control mode or CMV mode) or a pressure-controlled mode. This is an extremely uncomfortable mode of ventilation for the patient and requires complete patient-ventilator synchrony. Therefore, in utilizing an inverse-ratio mode of ventilation, it is often required that you deeply sedate +/- employ muscle relaxants in these patients.

NUTRITIONAL SUPPORT

Nutritional support is extremely important and often not given enough emphasis. Use the enteral route whenever possible. After major surgery or the onset of sepsis, metabolic requirements increase dramatically. Requirements peak in 3–5 days. If the patient is unable to eat, start enteral feedings or TPN as soon as possible after the initial insult. Even though enteral feeding increases the possibility of aspiration, it is preferred over TPN, because it tends to maintain the intestinal epithelium and its natural defenses against bacteria. Enteral feeding is contraindicated in only 2 cases:
1) patients with severe pancreatitis with associated abdominal pain
2) prior to, and just after, abdominal surgery (even in this situation, surgeons will feed immediately post-op when using a jejunostomy)

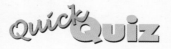

Quick Quiz

1) What are the 2 categories of actions you keep in mind when adjusting a ventilator?

2) When should you use PEEP?

3) A patient with severe COPD is placed on the ventilator. She suddenly becomes hypotensive. What steps should you follow to stabilize her?

4) What is "inverse ratio ventilation," and when is it used?

5) What is the best method to provide nutrition for a mechanically ventilated patient?

6) What is refeeding syndrome and how do you prevent it?

Otherwise, feed enterally!

With enteral feeding, you decrease the risk of aspiration and pneumonia by keeping the head of the bed elevated ≥ 30°. Position of head is more important than where the feeding tube is placed (e.g., pre- vs. post-pyloric).

Refeeding syndrome occurs when severely malnourished patients are fed high carbohydrate loads. These patients develop low total body levels of phosphorus, magnesium, and potassium. With refeeding syndrome:

• There is a dramatic increase in circulating insulin levels and a resulting swift uptake of glucose, K^+, phosphate, and magnesium into the cells—with a precipitous drop of these agents in the serum. The resulting severe hypophosphatemia causes heart and respiratory failure, rhabdomyolysis, RBC and WBC dysfunction, seizures, and coma.

• The body also begins to retain fluid (unknown why), and heart failure may result.

Prevent refeeding syndrome by starting the feeding of severely malnourished patients slowly, and aggressively give phosphate, potassium, and magnesium supplementation.

PULMONARY ARTERY CATHETERIZATION

Overview

Right heart and pulmonary artery catheterization is done with a balloon-floated (Swan-Ganz) catheter.

• As the catheter is introduced—usually via the internal jugular vein—take pressure readings of the central venous pressure, right atrial (0–8 mmHg nl), right ventricle (0–8 enddiastolic; 15–30 systolic), and pulmonary artery (3–12 enddiastolic; 15–30 systolic) pressures.

• When the catheter has been flow-directed to a small pulmonary artery, the balloon at the tip can be temporarily fully inflated, and the reading (wedge pressure) is the dampened left atrial pressure (LAP—normals are: A wave: 3–15; V wave: 3–12; mean: 5–12 mmHg). LAP is a reflection of LVEDP in a patient with a normal mitral valve. LVEDP is a reflection of LV preload (assuming compliance is not changed). This LVEDP is the all-important indicator of the likelihood for LVF and pulmonary edema.

Thermal-dilution cardiac output (CO) is done by injecting a known temperature (usually 32°F but may be room temperature) and known volume of water proximal to the tip of the PA catheter, then measuring temperature at the tip of the catheter. These values are put into a formula that calculates CO, taking into account temperature at the tip, and the volume and temperature of the fluid (D5W) injected. The greater the difference in temperature, the higher the CO—because more warm blood is mixed with the fluid injected from the proximal catheter port before it reaches the distal tip.

Mixed venous oxygen saturation (SVO_2). This is the last measurement of venous blood before it gets oxygenated. Normally, the SVO_2 is 78%. This number drops as the global tissue oxygen debt increases. If it gets too low, you must boost delivery of O_2 to the tissues (increase O_2 sat, cardiac output, or Hgb concentration—discussed at beginning of this section).

Systemic Vascular Resistance (SVR) measurement reflects vascular tone: vasodilated vs. vasoconstricted.
$$SVR = (MAP - CVP)\ 80/CO$$
(MAP=mean art press; CVP = central venous press)

Complications of PA Catheterization:

Establishing central venous access can cause unintentional puncture of nearby arteries, bleeding, neuropathy, air embolism, and pneumothorax.

Advancing the catheter may cause dysrhythmias, which are usually transitory but may be persistent. Cardiac advancement can cause RHB and, in a patient with LHB, this may result in complete heart block.

Catheter residing in the pulmonary artery may cause pulmonary artery rupture (53% mortality), venous thrombosis, thrombophlebitis, pulmonary embolism, and pulmonary infarction.

The majority of ICU physicians believe PA catheterization is helpful in select groups of critically ill patients. Even so, despite over 30 years of use, there is little proof that Swan-Ganz catheters have improved patient outcomes. Indeed, in a review of PA catheterization (Conners, et al. JAMA 1996) evaluating outcomes (survival, ICU and total length of stay, costs) in patients at 5 teaching hospitals, each of the outcomes was worse for the patients undergoing PA catheterization! One explanation has been that perhaps the hemodynamic information supplied by the PA catheter was not acted on optimally. The outcome:

1) A large, multi-center, prospective, randomized, controlled trial is ongoing.

2) You should weigh the risks and benefits carefully for each patient.

3) Improved training and credentialing is being initiated.

notes

Optional devices: Trials/development is ongoing of noninvasive hemodynamic monitoring, such as echocardiography, tissue tonometry, and surface impedance plethysmography.

Know the following text and know Table 3-9:
Notes:
1) Hallmark of hypovolemia: low wedge pressure. This low LV preload → low stroke volume → low CO (once HR is maxed out; CO=HR x stroke volume) → high SVR. Treat by giving fluid.
2) Hallmark of cardiogenic shock: low CO (i.e., the pump ain't working) → high wedge pressure (pump backs up) and increased SVR.
3) Hallmark of distributive shock: loss of SVR → initially low wedge pressure → initially have high CO (e.g., "warm" septic shock), which becomes low with shock progression. Treat septic shock by:
   a. removing source,
   b. giving fluids, and
   c. giving vasopressors (to increase SVR).
   Know that this is the only subset of shock in which the SVR is low. In all other cases, the high SVR is the only thing keeping blood pressure high enough to sustain life.
4) Hallmark of obstructive shock: low filling pressure → low wedge pressure → low CO → high SVR. Treat by resolving the obstructive problem +/- fluids.

Table 3-9: PA Catheterizaton and Shock

PA Catheterization Review: Hemodynamic Subsets of Shock			
TYPE	CO	Wedge	SVR
Hypovolemic	Low	LOW	High
Cardiogenic	LOW	High	High
Distributive†	High-Nl-Low	Low	LOW
Obstructive‡	Low	Low	High

†Distributive as seen in sepsis, spinal, and anaphylactic shock--have total loss of SVR.
‡Obstructive as in massive PE or tension pneumothorax. From John Morrissey, MD

By the way, tension pneumothorax causes torsion of the heart and increased intrathoracic pressure. Torsion of the heart → twisting the great vessels, thereby causing obstruction. Increased intrathoracic pressure → decreases venous return, also causing obstruction.

SLEEP APNEA
OVERVIEW

Sleep apnea is defined as a cessation of airflow of > 10 sec (usually 20–30 sec) during sleep. It becomes clinically significant at 10–15 episodes per hour, and severe cases may have > 40 per hr. Oxygen saturation usually decreases by > 4% during the apneic episodes. The 2 main classes of sleep apnea are central and obstructive, although it can also be a combination of the 2.

By definition, patients with sleep apnea have daytime hypersomnolence. When severe, pulmonary hypertension/cor pulmonale (from the chronic hypoxia) and personality changes may develop.

Systolic hypertension: An episode of sleep apnea typically causes a rapid transient increase in blood pressure—right at the end of the apneic episode. Some have wondered if this carries forward to daytime systolic hypertension, and it has been found that those with sleep apnea are slightly more likely to have systolic hypertension (odds ratio = 2). More studies are needed to better define the relationship. There have been no studies to determine how many of those with hypertension have sleep apnea.

Diagnosis is confirmed only by polysomnography (sleep study). The patient is hooked up to multiple electronic gadgets (ECG, EEG, EMG, oximeter, tidal CO_2 recorder) during sleep. Presence or absence of inspiratory effort during the apneic episode differentiates between obstructive and central apnea. O_2 desaturation to < 85% or of > 4% are significant. The frequency of hypoxic apneic episodes determines the severity of the disease. Normal is < 5–10/hr, mild is 5–20/hr; moderate is 20–30/hr; and severe disease is > 30/hr (again, various definitions).

OSA

Obstructive sleep apnea (OSA) is sleep apnea occurring despite continuing ventilatory effort. The obstructive episode is usually followed by a loud snore. Patients have daytime hypersomnolence and snoring, and may have headaches, recent weight gains, and hypertension. It is frequently associated with an abnormal airway, myxedema, and obesity (but none of these, including obesity, is a necessary feature). Causes of an abnormal airway include tonsillar hypertrophy or lymphoma, micrognathia, acromegaly, goiter, and TMJ disease.

Pickwickian syndrome. Unlike most patients with obesity-related sleep apnea (obesity-hypoventilation syndrome), the "Pickwickian patients" not only have extreme daytime sleepiness, but also have hypoventilation (i.e., high PCO_2) while awake; it is considered a severe form of the obesity-hypoventilation syndrome. Again: All patients with Pickwickian syndrome have obstructive sleep apnea, but most patients with obesity-hypoventilation sleep apnea are not Pickwickian.

notes

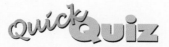

Treatment of OSA:

Treat the most persistent and significant OSA with either nCPAP or BiPAP. With nCPAP (nasal continuous positive airway pressure), air at constant pressure (5–15 cm H_2O) is supplied via a well-sealed nose mask. This "splints" the pharynx open at night. It is very effective. BiPAP (bi-level positive airway pressure) is similar, but can be used with a nasal or full face mask and allows independent adjustment for inspiratory and expiratory pressures. This improves comfort and compliance.

You can often treat mild-to-moderate OSA successfully with weight loss, avoiding alcohol/sedatives/hypnotics, and not sleeping in the supine position. Nasal and intraoral patency devices may also help.

Treat moderate OSA with uvulopalatopharyngoplasty and/or either nCPAP or BiPAP. Uvulopalatopharyngoplasty often eliminates the snoring but, overall, it cures only 50% of OSA. It is most effective in young, thin patients with mild-to-moderate obstructive sleep apnea and in those with certain specific sites of obstruction. It is sometimes used in severe sleep apnea to decrease the amount of PAP required.

The tricyclic protriptyline is used with varying success. Tracheostomy is effective treatment for severe OSA.

Obstructive sleep *hypopnea* is defined as a 30–50% decrease in airflow, > 15 episodes per hour, often with > 4% desat. Daytime symptoms are the same as those with obstructive sleep apnea.

CSA

Central sleep apnea (CSA) occurs in < 5% of sleep apnea patients. Cheyne-Stokes breathing is a type of central apnea and is usually seen with CNS disease, but it frequently occurs in healthy persons when they're in high altitudes for the first time, and it is also seen in CHF patients. Ondine's curse is a very rare syndrome, in which breathing is a voluntary function only.

Treatment of CSA: Avoid CNS depressants such as alcohol, sedatives, and hypnotics. Weight loss prn and avoid sleep deprivation.

Mild CSA treatment is not standardized. Try different therapies. Supplemental nighttime oxygen has been helpful for those with hypoxemia. Acetazolamide is often helpful; it causes a metabolic acidosis that stimulates a central compensatory response. Medroxyprogesterone appears to be effective only when there is waking hypercapnia. Nasal CPAP or even BiPAP may be useful, especially in those with CSA secondary to CHF.

Question: When do nocturnal O_2 desats occur without apnea? Answer: COPD/emphysema, kyphoscoliosis, and muscular dystrophy.

LUNG CANCER

NOTE

Lung cancer is the #2 cancer among men (after prostate) and the #2 cancer among white/American Indian/Alaskan native women (after breast; #3 in black and Hispanic women after breast and colorectal). Lung cancer is the leading cause of death in men and women (except Hispanic women in whom breast cancer is leading cause of death)!

85% of lung cancers are linked to smoking! The risk decreases for 15 years after smoking is stopped, until it returns to normal. Lung function also improves after smoking cessation, but not to normal.

RISK FACTORS FOR LUNG CANCER

With significant asbestos exposure alone, risk of lung cancer is 6 x normal; with smoking alone it is 10 x normal. With asbestos and smoking, the risk is 60 x normal (synergistic). Asbestos is associated with the 2 most common lung cancers: adenocarcinoma and squamous. There is also an increased incidence of lung cancer with uranium and nickel mining and exposure to hexavalent chromium and arsenic. Heavy doses of radon in underground miners are associated with lung cancer, but home/office exposure as a cause is controversial. Atmospheric pollution is a risk factor for lung cancer. Second-hand smoke (> 25 pack-years) increases the chance of lung cancer in persons < age 20. Non-filter cigarettes are worse than those with filters. There is a definite genetic factor in susceptibility.

Malignant mesothelioma is associated with asbestos, but not with smoking. It is usually considered pathognomonic for asbestos exposure. Note that the death rates from mesothelioma are lower for smokers than nonsmokers(!)...because the smokers often die of another lung cancer first! It usually presents with pleuritic chest pain and a unilateral hemorrhagic pleural effusion.

notes

Silica, when it causes silicosis, has a possible association with lung cancer.

TYPES OF LUNG CANCER

There are four major categories of cancer (shown with proportion of incidence):
1) Adenocarcinoma (1/3)   2) Squamous cell (1/3)
3) Small cell (1/4)   4) Large cell (1/5)
(hASSLe: 1/3, 1/3, 1/4, 1/5—Lung cancer is a "hASSLe"!).

Adenocarcinoma just beats out squamous cell as the most common lung cancer.
Squamous and small cell cancers are usually central lesions (S-S-SENTRAL). Adeno and large cell are peripheral.

Adenocarcinoma is usually peripheral and is usually found incidentally. Adenocarcinoma metastasizes early, especially to the CNS, adrenals, and bones. It usually presents as a solitary nodule. A "bronchoalveolar carcinoma" is a subclass of adenocarcinoma that may produce a large amount of frothy sputum; it has the least association with smoking and a strong association with pulmonary scars (as in idiopathic pulmonary fibrosis). In severe cases, the chest x-ray is indistinguishable from ARDS.

Squamous cell cancer, unlike adenocarcinoma, does not metastasize early. It usually is a central/hilar lesion with local extension and often presents with obstructive symptoms (atelectasis, pneumonitis), and occasionally (7%) presents as a thick-walled (> 4 mm) cavitation. Squamous cell lung cancer is by far the most likely lung cancer to cavitate.

Small cell cancer (previously called oat cell) is extremely aggressive—80% of patients have metastases at the time of diagnosis—so its treatment is usually discussed separately from the others. Contrary to other lung cancers, cavitation never occurs. Small cell lung cancer can cause SIADH, ectopic ACTH production, and Eaton-Lambert (myasthenic) syndrome.

Large cell cancer is usually a peripheral lesion and tends to metastasize to the CNS and mediastinum (may cause hoarseness or SVC syndrome).
If there is a history of asbestos exposure, think of squamous cell cancer, adenocarcinoma, and mesothelioma.

SOLITARY PULMONARY NODULE

The "solitary pulmonary nodule" [Know!] is a nodule in the middle-to-lateral 1/3 of the lung, surrounded by normal parenchyma. Clinically, 35% are malignant.
Calcification of a solitary pulmonary nodule suggests it is benign. It is virtually always benign if the calcification is "popcorn" (hamartoma), laminated ("bulls eye" = granuloma), or has multiple punctate foci or dense central calcification.

In low-risk patients (e.g., age < 35 and a nonsmoker), just follow a solitary calcified nodule with chest x-rays q 3 months. It is considered benign if, after 2 years, there is no growth.

High-risk patients require a diagnosis. This can be accomplished using:
1) fine-needle aspiration (must be able to hit the center of the nodule; 10–15% risk of pneumothorax)
2) bronchoscopy (won't reach peripheral lesions)
3) open lung biopsy (can remove the nodule at the same time)
4) if nodules are > 1 cm diameter, 5-fluorodeoxyglucose + PET scan may also be able to sort out benign from malignant lesions.

PARANEOPLASTIC SYNDROMES

Paraneoplastic syndromes occur in ~ 2% of lung cancer patients [Know]:
• Hypercalcemia is associated with squamous cancer (think $sca^{++}mous!...?$). The calcium level is proportional to the tumor bulk. Hypercalcemia is seen less often in large cell (12%).

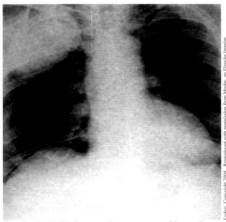
Image 3-19: Right apical carcinoma of bronchus (Pancoast tumour)

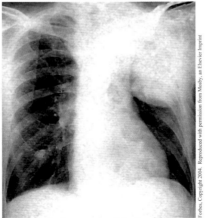
Image 3-20: Carcinoma of the bronchus with left upper lobe opacity

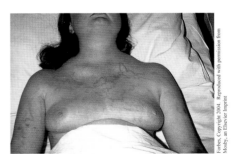
Image 3-21: Superior vena caval obstruction in bronchial carcinoma

notes

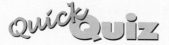

Quick Quiz

1) Which lung cancer is usually centrally located?

2) Which lung cancer is usually peripherally located?

3) Which lung cancer is most likely to cavitate?

4) A "popcorn" calcification on CXR is indicative of what?

5) Which lung cancer/s is/are most commonly associated with SIADH? With hypercalcemia? With gynecomastia? With hypertrophic pulmonary osteoarthropathy (HPO)?

6) Anterior mediastinotomy is useful for assessing what area of the chest?

7) What is generally the sequence for the diagnostic workup of lung cancer in a patient without palpable lymph nodes?

8) Which "T," which "N," and which "M" determines if a lung cancer is unresectable?

• SIADH, ectopic ACTH production, and Eaton-Lambert (myasthenic) syndrome are associated with small cell cancer (Wow, small cells do all that?). Example: A 65-year-old man presents with weakness that progresses throughout the day. Chest x-ray shows a central lung mass. What is the diagnosis? Answer: Small cell cancer (Eaton-Lambert syndrome).

• Gynecomastia is associated with large cell cancer (My, what large cells you have, er...sir! (...hey, this is the only iffy one in the entire book!))

• Hypertrophic pulmonary osteoarthropathy (HPO) is especially associated with adenocarcinoma, but it is seen in all three non-small cell types. With HPO, patients get clubbing and new bone formation on the long bones (these bones appear dense on x-rays). These patients often present with only painful ankles and clubbing.

Note: Diabetes insipidus is not a paraneoplastic syndrome. If a patient presents with this and a lung cancer, consider brain metastases!

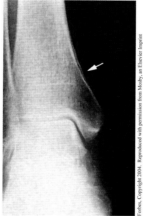

Image 3-22: Hypertrophic pulmonary osteoarthropathy

Forbes. Copyright 2004. Reproduced with permission from Mosby, an Elsevier Imprint

DIAGNOSIS AND STAGING OF LUNG CANCER

Diagnosis of lung cancer: Rule out extrathoracic spread. Generally, the initial workup does not require brain, bone, or liver-spleen scans. [Know]

First, do a careful H+P and lab tests—CBC, calcium, bilirubin, SGOT, SGPT, and alkaline phosphatase.

Then, follow up on any abnormal lab with the indicated nuclear or CT scans.

Then biopsy the scalene lymph nodes if any are palpable (90% yield!)

Then biopsy the cancer:

• Bronchoscopy usually is the procedure of choice. There is a 100% yield when the lesion is visible. There is also a good yield with peripheral lesions > 4 cm.

• Mediastinoscopy is accurate for assessing all areas of the mediastinum, except the lymph nodes in the aorto-pulmonary window (nodes affected by LUL tumors). It is considered the gold standard for assessing the mediastinum.

• Anterior mediastinotomy can assess the aortopulmonary window

• Needle-aspiration biopsy procedure is accurate for assessing all of the mediastinum. It is better than bronchoscopy in assessing peripheral lesions < 2 cm. To make the diagnosis of lymphoma, it is usually necessary to get more tissue than a needle biopsy can produce, so mediastinotomy/oscopy is the procedure of choice.

Staging—Tumor, node, mets description of lung cancer:

T indicates tumor size

• T1 is < or = 3 cm

• T2 is > 3 cm

• T3 means there is local extension—e.g., the tumor is invading the parietal pleura or chest wall. T3 is also used when the tumor is within 2 cm of the carina.

• T4 means the tumor has spread to the great vessels, trachea, mediastinum, esophagus—or patient has a malignant pleural effusion (nonresectable).

Lymph node involvement

• N0 = none

• N1 = hilar nodes

• N2 = mediastinal nodes

• N3 = contralateral nodes or ipsilateral supraclavicular (nonresectable)

Metastases

• M0 = absence

• M1= presence (nonresectable)

Table 3-10: Mediastinal Masses—Type vs. Location

Mediastinal Masses		
Anterior	**Middle**	**Posterior**
1) Thymoma 6) Aortic aneurysm 2) Thyroid tumor 7) Lymphoma 3) Parathyroid tumor 8) Thymus 4) Teratoma 9) Endocrine tumors 5) Lipoma	1) Lymphoma 2) Cysts 3) Lymphadenopathy 4) Aortic aneurysm 5) Hernia	1) Neurogenic tumors 2) Gastroenteric cysts 3) Esophageal lesions 4) Aortic aneurysms 5) Hernia

Of the primary mediastinal tumors:

20% = Cysts	10% = Lymphomas
20% = Neurogenic tumors	10% = Teratomas
20% = Thymomas*	20% = Miscellaneous

*Note that the thymomas are associated with autoimmune diseases such as myasthenia gravis.

Table 3-11: Findings in BAL

Bronchoalveolar Lavage	
Results	**Cause**
< 1% neutrophils; < 16% lymphocytes; no eosinophils	Normal findings
Increased neutrophils	Idiopathic pulmonary fibrosis (IPF), collagen vascular disease, asbestosis, suppurative infections, Wegener granulomatosis, ARDS
Increased lymphocytes	Hypersensitivity pneumonitis and sarcoidosis
Increased eosinophils	Chronic eosinophilic pneumonia, some ARDS
Diagnosis of specific types of pneumonias and other infectious diseases.	*95% sensitive for PCP in AIDS patients *CMV pneumonia (*inclusion bodies) *Disseminated TB or fungal infection *Diagnosing pneumonia in ARDS patients
Turbid, PAS-positive material	*Alveolar proteinosis
Langerhans cells	*Eosinophilic granulomatosis (histiocytosis x)
Bloody with a large amount of hemosiderin in the alveolar macrophages	*Diffuse alveolar hemorrhage
Hyperplastic and atypical type II pneumocytes	*Cytotoxic lung injury
"Foamy" changes with lamellar inclusions	*Amiodarone-induced disease
* In these, BAL results are sufficient for diagnosis.	

notes

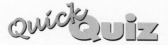

TREATMENT OF LUNG CANCER

[Know all of the following!]

Treatment of non-small cell lung cancer: The specific cell type of the non-small cell cancer makes little difference in survival. Stage I is treated with surgery and stage II with radical surgery. Radical surgery is also occasionally performed for Stage III if the nodal disease is ipsilateral. Radiation therapy is indicated for bone and CNS mets, but is palliative only; it also helps with large-volume hemoptysis, obstructive pneumonitis, and superior vena caval (SVC) syndrome.

Thoracotomy is the only treatment that can cure lung cancer. It is especially useful for small, central lesions and to rule out lymphoma. Surgical resection for a cure is possible only in the non-small cell types, and only if the cancer is diagnosed when localized to thorax and the lobar lymph nodes.

Do not do surgery if extrathoracic mets exist (M1), or if the cancer has spread to supraclavicular lymph nodes or contra-lateral nodes (N3), or is T4. Surgery is also virtually never indicated if there is involvement of the mediastinal nodes (N2), pharyngeal nerve, or phrenic nerve (see next for the only exception). The borderline cases when surgery may be indicated include the following stage IIIa tumors:
- when there is a solitary ipsilateral mediastinal lymph node involved, and
- tumors within 2 cm of the carina, but not involving it (17% 5-year survival).

Remember: Stages T4 and N3 are not resectable.

For small cell cancer, use chemotherapy, radiation therapy, or occasionally adjuvant surgery. Because of the poor prognosis, all treatment for small cell cancer is only palliative.

Chemotherapy and radiation treatment are generally considered only palliative, although some studies suggest a benefit if they are used as adjuvant treatment.

Pre-op contraindications:
- myocardial infarction within the last 3 months (20% die); within last 6 months is a relative contraindication
- uncontrolled major arrhythmias
- severe pulmonary hypertension
- pre-op hypoxia
- pre-op CO_2 retention
- pre-op $FEV_1/FVC < 80\%$
- pre-op $FEV_1 < 1$ L (1.1–2.4 still risky; > 2.5 will permit a pneumonectomy)
- predicted post-op $FEV_1/FVC < 40\%$ or $FEV_1 < 1L$

An alternative to PFTs in this situation is a V/Q quantitative lung scan—or the perfusion part (Q) of the scan.

SVC SYNDROME

Superior Vena Caval Syndrome. Most (75–85%) are due to bronchogenic carcinoma—especially small cell. The other cases are usually caused by lymphoma. Rarely, it is the result of an aortic aneurysm. SVC can also be caused by mediastinal fibrotic processes—e.g., histoplasmosis, TB, and select drugs such as methysergide.

MEDIASTINAL MASSES

[Know Table 3-10.]

BRONCHOALVEOLAR LAVAGE

[Know Table 3-11.]

APPENDIX A

GOING DEEPER INTO THE A-a GRADIENT.

I didn't want to wear you out on this topic in the main text, but one more question pops up. What about changes in barometric pressure? Does it change the alveolar O_2 much (and hence, your P_aO_2)? The quick answer is "no." The slower answer follows…

Okay, 1 problem is that the barometric pressure is given in inchesHg instead of mmHg. 29.92 inchesHg is standard atmospheric pressure. This is equal to the 760 mmHg (or 760 Torr) that we use in the respiratory equations.

One source of confusion is that, say, at 6,500 ft, the normal barometric pressure is ~ 23.4 inchesHg, but the weatherman and all barometers will say 29.92. Why in the world is this? It is because all the barometers are referenced to sea level so weathermen and pilots can understand the pressure without knowing the altitude at which each reading was taken.

notes

Anyway, the atmospheric pressure changes by only 1 inch Hg or 25 mmHg or so normally, which translates to the equivalent of about a thousand feet of difference in elevation. Even a category 5 hurricane, which has a central pressure of about 27 inchesHg, causes a pressure drop equivalent to only a 2000 ft elevation change. So don't worry about changes in atmospheric pressure, because large changes in elevation are much more relevant. Even so, if you have a COPD patient on the slippery slope of the oxygen dissociation curve (with a low S_aO_2 and very low P_aO_2) who tells you he feels worse just before a big rainstorm (when barometric pressure drops), believe what you hear!

One of your patients with ILD wants to know if it is okay to take a flight on an airliner. How do you use these formulas and tables to help with your decision?

Hopefully, you already know what his A-a gradient is. You also know that all airliners are pressurized to maintain at least an 8,000 ft equivalent air pressure inside the cabin. You see from the chart that this level is ~ 560 mmHg. You plug this into the alveolar oxygen formula with a proportionately decreased water vapor pressure. So instead of

$$[(760-47) \times .209], \text{ we have } [(560-35) \times .209] = 110$$

Subtract this patient's A-a O_2 difference, and you have a good feel for what his P_aO_2 will be without supplemental oxygen. You can then check the O_2 saturation curve and see if the Hgb saturation is going to be sufficient. If need be, you can prescribe supplemental oxygen.

COPD patients do not have a pure diffusion problem, but you can use this same method to approximate the change from baseline that going up to an equivalent 8,000 ft altitude will cause.

Elevation in feet	mmHg (Torr)	Inches Hg	psi
-3,280	854.3318	33.63472	16.52
-1,640	806.2369	31.74124	15.59
0	760.2105	29.9292	14.7
820	737.4559	29.03336	14.26
1,640	716.2528	28.1986	13.85
2,461	695.0496	27.36384	13.44
3,281	673.8465	26.52908	13.03
4,101	653.6776	25.73504	12.64
4,921	634.0259	24.96136	12.26
5,742	614.8914	24.20804	11.89
6,562	596.274	23.47508	11.53
8,202	560.0735	22.04988	10.83
9,843	525.9416	20.70612	10.17
11,483	493.3611	19.42344	9.54
13,123	462.3321	18.20184	8.94
14,764	433.3717	17.06168	8.38
16,404	405.4456	15.96224	7.84
18,045	379.071	14.92388	7.33
19,685	354.2478	13.9466	6.85
21,325	330.4589	13.01004	6.39

notes

The following material is to assist you in integrating the information you have just reviewed in this section. These are purposely NOT Board-style questions since they are meant to cover a lot of material in minimal space. MedStudy does have Board-style Q&A products separately available in book and software formats.

TRUE/FALSE

1) Respiratory Physiology:
   A. The "blue bloater" and the "pink puffer" are both chronic hypoxics, although the pink puffer does not retain CO_2 and the blue bloater does.
   B. Decreased diffusion is the main cause of hypoxemia in chronic lung disease.
   C. The A-a O_2 difference is increased in all causes of hypoxemia, except hypoventilation and low F_iO_2.
   D. Emphysema and interstitial lung disease cause a decreased DLCO.
   E. The total lung capacity can easily be determined by spirometry.
   F. Most of the information we get from flow-volume loops is determined by where the graph intersects on the abscissa.

   [A=T, B=F (decreased diffusion is a minor component), C=T, D=T, E=F, F=F (it is determined by the shape and size of the loop)]

2) Obstructive lung disease:
   A. Some asthma is IgA-mediated.
   B. Most asthmatics have a nonspecific airway hyperresponsivity.
   C. The most effective treatment for asthma is steroids.
   D. Theophylline is recommended as adjunctive treatment in acute asthma.
   E. Ipratropium may work better than beta-agonists in patients with COPD.
   F. Only O_2 and smoking cessation improve survival of COPD patients.
   G. Cromolyn sodium is a mild bronchodilator.
   H. Bullae are found in the apices of the lungs of smokers with emphysema and in the bases of patients with alpha-1 antitrypsin deficiency.
   I. There is no treatment for alpha-1 antitrypsin deficiency.
   J. Because the amount of emphysema best correlates with the amount of decreased airflow seen in COPD patients, the best prognostic indicator in COPD is FEV_1.
   K. In nonsmokers, the average decrease in FEV_1 is ~ 15–30 cc per year; whereas in smokers, it is 50–100 cc per year.
   L. A CO_2 retainer should never be given > 2 liters O_2 by nasal cannula.

[A=F (IgE), B=T, C=F (the most effective treatment is removal of known causative agents, then steroids), D=F, E=T, F=T, G=F, H=T, I=F (treatment *is* IV alpha-1 antiprotease or lung transplant), J=T, K=F (In *both* it is 15–30cc/year! Only a minority of smokers develop COPD), L=F (should be as needed to maintain an O_2 sat of 90%)]

3) Interstitial Lung Disease:
   A. Interstitial lung disease classically shows a restrictive pattern.
   B. Hypersensitivity pneumonitis should be considered in patients with a history of recurrent pneumonias.
   C. Asbestosis generally requires < 5 years exposure to asbestos.
   D. Silicosis and berylliosis tend to affect the upper lobes; whereas asbestosis affects the lower lobes.
   E. Although > 30% of patients with rheumatoid arthritis get ILD, the most common lung problem in RA is pleurisy.
   F. Patients may get ILD from rheumatoid arthritis or from gold or methotrexate treatment for rheumatoid arthritis.
   G. Both rheumatoid arthritis and scleroderma are associated with exposure to silica, and both have increased incidence of bronchogenic carcinoma.
   H. In sarcoidosis, bronchial alveolar lavage will show a helper-to-suppressor lymphocyte ratio of < 1.
   I. If a patient with sarcoidosis also has erythema nodosum, he/she has a better prognosis.
   J. Lymphangioleiomyomatosis occurs in premenopausal women only.
   K. Eosinophilic granuloma causes granulomatous bone lesions.
   L. The ANCA is used to confirm the diagnosis of Wegener granulomatosis.
   M. Of the vasculitides that cause ILD, polyarteritis nodosa is the only one that is not granulomatous.
   N. Hemoptysis can be seen in ILD secondary to SLE, Wegener granulomatosis, Goodpasture syndrome, or idiopathic pulmonary hemosiderosis.
   O. ABPA is associated with a very high IgA.

   [A=T, B=T, C=F (>10 years), D=T, E=T, F=T, G=T, H=F (> 4; hypersensitivity pneumonitis is < 1), I=T, J=T, K=F (*lytic* bone lesions), L=F (ANCA is an *adjunctive* test; nasal biopsy or open lung biopsy confirms the diagnosis), M=T, N=T, O=F (IgE)]

4) Pulmonary Hypertension:
   A. In primary pulmonary hypertension, patients may have dyspnea, but they never have chest pain.
   B. Heart-lung transplant is the only long-term solution.

   [A=F (they have dyspnea *and* chest pain with exercise), B=F (both heart-lung and single-lung transplants are possible long-term solutions.]

5) Pleural Effusions:
   A. Chylous pleural effusions are defined as effusions with a triglyceride level > 50 mg/dl.
   B. A pleural fluid glucose of 80 suggests TB, 60 suggests cancer and empyema, and < 30 suggests RA.
   C. Pleural biopsy is the procedure of choice in diagnosing a pleural-based malignancy.
   D. Pleural biopsy is the procedure of choice if a pleural effusion is thought to be caused by tuberculosis.
   E. Relief of dyspnea after thoracentesis is due to an increase in the intrathoracic volume.

   [A=F (> 115), B=T, C=F (pleurocentesis is quicker and equally good), D=T (much better results than pleurocentesis), E=F (decrease!!)]

6) Pneumonia:
   A. Viral pneumonias are the most common type of nosocomial pneumonia.
   B. If a patient's pneumococcal pneumonia is bacteremic, mortality is 10%.
   C. Salmon-pink sputum is suggestive of *Staph aureus* pneumonia.
   D. A 3rd generation cephalosporin or vancomycin is the treatment of choice in *Staph aureus* pneumonia.
   E. *Legionella* is the cause of pneumonia in 25% of patients hospitalized for community-acquired pneumonias.
   F. With influenza A and B, age > 65 years is only a slight risk factor for increased mortality.
   G. A positive tuberculin skin test is defined as >10 mm of induration.
   H. The typical treatment for pulmonary tuberculosis is 18 weeks of INH, rifampin, and PZA.
   I. INH must be given for 12 months in the prophylaxis of tuberculosis.
   J. After aspirating, a patient should be started on antibiotics if any chest x-ray changes develop.
   K. Best results are obtained in a sputum C + S if the specimen contains > 25 WBCs per low-power field.

   [A=F (bacterial!: Gram-neg > *Staph=Strep=H. flu*), B=F (30%), C=T, D=F (1st gen ceph, penicillinase-resistant PCN, or vancomycin), E=F (1–5%), F=F (large risk factor), G=F (The current recommendations take into account the clinical suspicion of TB. If there is no clinical suspicion of TB, a positive skin test {5TU-PPD-Mantoux} requires 15 mm of induration. If there is a strong clinical suspicion of TB {close contacts, suggestive chest x-ray, HIV patients}, a positive skin test requires only 5 mm of induration), H=F (The usual treatment is 2 months of 4-drug therapy {INH + rifampin + PZA and either ethambutol or streptomycin}, followed by 4 months of INH and rifampin—if sensitive.), I=F (9 months is standard for almost all patients), J= F (no antibiotics are indicated until a fever develops, because usually only a chemical pneumonitis develops with aspiration), K=T]

7) Immunosuppressed patients:
   A. CMV is the most common cause of fever after transplant.
   B. Tuberculosis is usually very effectively treated in AIDS patients.
   C. Unlike *Aspergillus*, *Cryptococcus* is not normally found in sputum, so *Cryptococcus neoformans* in the sputum means infection.
   D. Patients with lymphoma are at especially high risk for pulmonary mucormycosis.

   [A=T, B=T, C=T, D=F (Patients with leukemia are at high risk.)]

8) Noninfectious infiltrates:
   A. Only drugs that have cytotoxic reactions cause atypia of the Type II alveolar cells.
   B. Methotrexate is the most common cause of cytotoxic lung reactions.

   [A=T, B=F (methotrexate is the most common cause of *non*-cytotoxic lung reactions; bleomycin is the most common cytotoxic cause)]

9) Critical care:
   A. Tidal volume is usually greatly increased in ARDS patients.
   B. Corticosteroids are always included as adjunctive treatment for ARDS.
   C. A septic patient may have a normal P_aO_2 and still have abnormal O_2 uptake by the tissues—contributing to multi-organ failure.
   D. Hypophosphatemia decreases diaphragmatic contractility in addition to shifting the O_2 saturation curve to the left.
   E. Tracheostomy is indicated after 1 week of intubation, if needed, to decrease airway resistance during weaning.
   F. In ventilator patients with severe COPD, the respiratory rate must be slower than normal to prevent progressive air trapping.
   G. PEEP should not be used with focal lung disease.

   [A=F (decreased), B=F (corticosteroids may be useful only in ARDS caused by *fat* emboli), C=T, D=T, E=F (tracheostomy is done after 2–3 weeks of intubation, barring contraindication; it is never done to decrease airway resistance during weaning), F=T, G=T]

10) Pulmonary Embolism and DVT:
   A. Pulmonary angiogram is generally required to confirm the diagnosis of a high probability V/Q scan.
   B. If a PE is suspected and there are no contraindications to anticoagulants, the patient should always be started on heparin before the V/Q scan is done.
   C. In adjusted-dose heparin given after a PE, the dose is adjusted to maintain the PTT to at least 1.5 times normal.
   D. Warfarin should not be given to pregnant patients.
   E. Phlegmasia cerulea dolens (complete obstruction of the venous outflow of a limb) is very suggestive of malignancy.
   F. Risk of PE (in an unprophylaxed patient) is higher for knee replacement than for hip replacement.
   G. Anticoagulants may be used sparingly in patients undergoing neurosurgery, eye surgery, and open prostatectomy.

[A=F (A high probability scan should be treated; pulmonary angiogram is used only after a low-moderate scan when the index of suspicion is high), B=T, C=T, D=T, E=T (50% have malignancy!), F=T (knee:70%; hip: 50%), G=F (they should never be used in these surgeries!)]

11) Sleep Apnea:
   A. Apnea is defined as halting of breathing > 10 seconds.
   B. Sleep apnea becomes clinically significant at > 5 episodes/hour.
   C. Most patients with obesity-related sleep apnea are not Pickwickian, because they do not have daytime hypoventilation.
   D. Nasal CPAP is highly effective treatment for moderate obstructive sleep apnea.

   [A=T, B=F (> 10–15 per hour), C=T, D=T]

12) Lung Cancer:
   A. 1/2 of all lung cancer is linked directly to smoking.
   B. With asbestos exposure alone, the risk of lung cancer is 6 x normal. With smoking, it is 10 x normal. With asbestos and smoking, it is 16 x normal (additive).
   C. Silica has no association with lung cancer.
   D. Squamous and small cell lung cancers are usually peripheral lesions.
   E. 80% of patients with small cell cancer have metastases at time of diagnosis.
   F. Solitary pulmonary nodules are virtually always benign if they are calcified.
   G. Bronchoscopy is the procedure of choice in diagnosing lung cancer when there is a peripheral lesion > 4 cm.
   H. Mediastinoscopy is the gold standard for assessing all lesions in the mediastinum.

   [A=F (85%!), B=F (smoking + asbestos causes a 60x N increased risk of cancer; synergistic), C=F (silicosis has a possibly slight association with lung cancer), D=F (central lesions), E=T, F=T, G=T, H=F (all except those in the aortopulmonary window)]

SINGLE BEST ANSWER

13) A. V/Q mismatch.
   B. RL shunting.
   C. Hypoventilation.
   D. Decreased diffusion.

1. Main cause of hypoxemia in COPD.
2. Responds poorly to 100% O_2.
3. Always associated with an elevated PCO_2.
4. Main cause of hypoxemia in ARDS.

   [1 (A) 2 (B) 3 (C) 4 (B)]

14) Bronchoalveolar lavage
   A. PAS-positive material.
   B. Langerhans cells.
   C. Bloody with hemosiderin.
   D. Atypical type II pneumocytes.
   E. 5% neutrophils.
   F. 25% lymphocytes.
   G. 10% lymphocytes.
   H. Foamy changes with lamellar inclusions.
   I. High eosinophils.

1. Diffuse alveolar hemorrhage.
2. Normal.
3. Idiopathic pulmonary fibrosis.
4. Eosinophilic granulomatosis (Histiocytosis X).
5. Chronic eosinophilic pneumonia.
6. Sarcoidosis.
7. Asbestosis.
8. Amiodarone-induced lung disease.
9. Alveolar proteinosis.
10. Hypersensitivity pneumonitis.
11. Collagen vascular disease.
12. Cytotoxic lung disease.

   [1 (C) 2 (G) 3 (E) 4 (B) 5 (I) 6 (F) 7 (E) 8 (H) 9 (A) 10 (F) 11(E) 12 (D)]

15) Flow volume loops

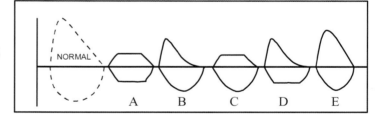

1. Restrictive lung disease.
2. Tracheal stenosis.
3. Obstructive lung disease.
4. Vocal cord paralysis.
5. Intrathoracic tracheomalacia.
6. Goiter.

   [1 (E) 2 (A) 3 (B) 4 (D; may be variable) 5 (C) 6 (D; as in vocal cord paralysis and extrathoracic tracheomalacia)]

16) FEV_1/FVC
   A. 0.4
   B. 0.8

1. Normal.
2. Restrictive lung disease.
3. Obstructive lung disease.

   [1 (B) 2 (B) 3 (A)]

17) A. Increases theophylline clearance.
     B. Decreases theophylline clearance.
     C. Neither.

1. Cigarette smoking.
2. Flu vaccine.
3. Erythromycin.
4. Doxycycline.
5. Ciprofloxacin.
6. Rifampin.
7. Cimetidine.
8. Phenobarbital.
9. Liver failure.
10. Metoclopramide.

[1 (A) 2 (B) 3 (B) 4 (C) 5 (B) 6 (A) 7 (B) 8 (A) 9 (B) 10 (C)]

18) A. Beta-agonists.
     B. Anticholinergics.
     C. Theophylline.
     D. Glucocorticoids.
     E. Cromolyn sodium.

1. Works best in patients with COPD.
2. Potentiates beta-agonists.
3. First choice for acute exacerbation of asthma.
4. Ipratropium.
5. Antiasthma medication with the least side effects.

[1 (B) 2 (D) 3 (A) 4 (B) 5 (E)]

19) A. Smoking
     B. Alpha-1 antitrypsin deficiency
     C. Both
     D. Neither

1. Panacinar emphysema.
2. Centroacinar emphysema.
3. Decreased lung compliance.
4. Bullae in the lung apices.
5. Bullae in the lung bases.
6. Causes chronic bronchitis.
7. Decreased elastic recoil.

[1 (B) 2 (A) 3 (D) 4 (A) 5 (B) 6 (A) 7 (C)]

20) Best diagnostic test:
     A. Bronchiectasis.
     B. Pulmonary hypertension.
     C. Wegener granulomatosis.
     D. Pulmonary embolus.
     E. Hypersensitivity pneumonitis.
     F. Bleomycin lung toxicity.
     G. ARDS vs. CHF.

1. Right heart catheterization.
2. Pulmonary artery wedge pressure.
3. Transbronchial lung biopsy.
4. High-resolution CT (HRCT) or MDCT.
5. History.

6. Pulmonary angiogram.
7. Nasal membrane biopsy.

[1 (B) 2 (G) 3 (F) 4 (A or D) 5 (E) 6 (D) 7 (C)]

21) Interstitial lung diseases
     A. Alveolar proteinosis.
     B. Acute bronchopulmonary aspergillosis.
     C. SLE.
     D. Lymphangioleiomyomatosis.
     E. Asbestosis.
     F. Rheumatoid arthritis.
     G. Scleroderma (Systemic sclerosis).
     H. Berylliosis.
     I. Hypersensitivity pneumonitis.
     J. Allergic granulomatosis of Churg-Strauss.
     K. Idiopathic pulmonary fibrosis.
     L. Byssinosis.

1. Increased surfactant.
2. Pneumothorax; chylous pleural effusions.
3. Thermophilic actinomycetes.
4. Orthopneic dyspnea; affects lungs and pleura.
5. +ANA in 1/3, +RF in 1/5; no systemic changes.
6. Necrobiotic nodules.
7. Very high serum IgE.
8. Asthma and eosinophilia.
9. Hilar adenopathy.
10. Fibrosis of the lung bases.
11. "Monday chest tightness."
12. Pulmonary artery hypertension.

[1 (A) 2 (D) 3 (I) 4 (C) 5 (K) 6 (F) 7 (B) 8 (J and B; oops! this is supposed to be single best answer.) 9 (H) 10 (E; other causes of fibrosis of the lung bases: sarcoidosis, collagen vascular diseases, and IPF. Fibrosis of the upper lung fields: TB, silicosis, fungal diseases, eosinophilic granuloma, and chronic hypersensitivity pneumonitis) 11 (L) 12 (G)]

22) Pleural effusions
     A. Rheumatoid arthritis.
     B. Drug-induced lupus.
     C. Chylous effusions.
     D. Transudative values.
     E. Malignant effusion.
     F. SLE.
     G. Pseudochylous effusion.
     H. Exudative values.
     I. None of the above.

1. Glucose 25.
2. Triglycerides >115.
3. ANA positive, anti-histone positive.
4. White color clears with centrifugation.
5. LDH 135; T. protein ratio 0.4; glucose 85.
6. Examination of the fluid is as good as a pleural biopsy.
7. ANA positive, anti-ds-DNA positive.
8. Triglycerides < 75.
9. LDH 210; T. protein ratio 0.6; glucose 85.
10. LDH 250; T. protein ratio 0.4; glucose 65.

[1 (A) 2 (C) 3 (B) 4 (I) 5 (D) 6 (E) 7 (F) 8 (I; < 50 for pseudo-chylous) 9 (H) 10 (E)]

23) Pneumonias
    A. *Klebsiella*.
    B. *H. influenzae*.
    C. Q fever.
    D. Histoplasmosis.
    E. Tularemia.
    F. Coccidioidomycosis.
    G. PCP.

1. Exposure to cattle or sheep.
2. Immunoglobulin deficiency.
3. Patient with AIDS.
4. Patient skins animals.
5. Erythema nodosum.
6. Nursing home patient.
7. Mississippi and Ohio River valleys.

[1 (C) 2 (B; also *S. pneumonia*, *Moraxella*, and meningococcus) 3 (G) 4 (E) 5 (F; and travel to the Southwestern U.S.) 6 (A) 7 (D)]

24) Pneumonias: diagnosis
    A. KOH.
    B. IgM.
    C. Direct immunofluorescence (DIF).
    D. CIE.
    E. Coagglutination.
    F. Cold agglutinins.

1. RSV.
2. *Mycoplasma*.
3. *Legionella*.
4. *Coccidioides*.
5. Influenza A.

[1 (C) 2 (B) 3 (C; also urinary antigen for *Legionella*) 4 (A; also complement fixation titers) 5 (C)]

25) Primary immunodeficiencies and pneumonias
    A. Humoral deficiency alone.
    B. Cell-mediated deficiency alone.
    C. Decreased neutrophils.
    D. Combined cell-mediated and humoral deficiency.

1. AIDS.
2. Susceptible to viral infections.
3. Seen in AML and CML.
4. Susceptible to Gram-negative organisms, *Staph*, and fungi.
5. Susceptible to encapsulated organisms (*H. flu*, *Strep*, Meningococcus).
6. Seen in patients with lymphoma, uremia, post-transplant.

[1 (D; these patients mainly have cell-mediated deficiency but also have abnormal Ig production) 2 (B; also PCP, TB, fungus, *Legionella*, and *Nocardia*) 3 (C) 4 (C) 5 (A; as are patients with actual or effective asplenia—e.g., SS—or abnormal complement.) 6 (B; also patients receiving corticosteroids and alkylating agents)]

26) Noninfectious lung infiltrates
    A. Hemorrhagic infiltrates.
    B. Cytotoxic lung reaction.
    C. Noncytotoxic lung reaction.
    D. Leukemic infiltrates.
    E. Leukostatic infiltrates.
    F. None of the above.

1. Gold.
2. SLE.
3. AML.
4. Bleomycin.
5. ALL.
6. Radiation therapy.
7. Methotrexate.
8. Goodpasture.

[1 (C) 2 (A) 3 (A,E) 4 (B) 5 (D; rare) 6 (F; this is direct injury usually occurring within 6 months of treatment) 7 (C) 8 (A)]

27) Most common PE prophylaxis method:
    A. UF IV heparin.
    B. Xa inhibition with LMWH or fondaparinux
    C. External pneumatic compression.
    D. Coumadin.

1. Hip replacement.
2. Knee replacement.
3. Pneumonia patient.
4. 45-year-old undergoing abdominal surgery.
5. Neurosurgery.

[1 (B is most common; also warfarin with INR 2–3) 2 (B; less common; same as in previous answer) 3 (B; LMWH or low-dose heparin SQ—LMWH preferred) 4 (B; LMWH +/-/or graduated compression stockings along with early mobilization) 5 (C; LMWH may be started 48 hours after surgery)]

28) Lung cancers: paraneoplastic syndromes; associations.
    A. Squamous cell carcinoma.
    B. Adenocarcinoma.
    C. Small cell carcinoma.
    D. Large cell carcinoma.
    E. None of the above.

Name the single best association.
1. SIADH.
2. Gynecomastia.
3. Cavitation.
4. Hypertrophic pulmonary osteoarthropathy (HPO).
5. Metastasizes very early.
6. SVC syndrome.
7. ACTH production.
8. Hypercalcemia.

[1 (C) 2 (D) 3 (A) 4 (B; although it can be caused by any non-small cell ca) 5 (C) 6 (C; usually small cell, then large cell) 7 (C) 8 (A 25%; large cell 12%)]

SHORT-CASE SCENARIOS

29) 35-year-old woman complains of extreme dyspnea with mild exercise and occasional, associated chest pain. She has no significant past medical history. EKG shows right axis deviation. What will the chest x-ray show?
   A. Clear.
   B. CHF.
   C. Engorged pulmonary vasculature.
   D. LVH.
   E. RVH.

What are the usual treatments for this problem?
   A. Beta-blockers and anticoagulants.
   B. Calcium-channel blockers and beta-blockers.
   C. Calcium-channel blockers and anticoagulants.
   D. ACE inhibitors and beta-blockers.

[Diagnosis is primary pulmonary hypertension. First answer: E. Chest x-ray will show RVH and engorged pulmonary arteries (*not* the entire vasculature). Second answer: C. vasodilators (calcium-channel blockers), anticoagulants, and supplemental oxygen are the main therapies. Heart-lung transplant works, but is usually not feasible. IV prostacyclin (epoprostenol) is also beneficial.]

30) A 20-year-old asthmatic patient is found to have recurrent lung infiltrates and peripheral eosinophilia. A KOH stain of the sputum shows fungal elements with branching hyphae.

   A. This patient will have a high IgM.
   B. This patient with have a high IgE.
   C. The infiltrates are hemorrhagic.
   D. The asthma has nothing to do with the infiltrates.
   E. A workup for kidney dysfunction should be done.

[B. This patient has ABPA (acute bronchopulmonary aspergillosis). Remember, chronic eosinophilic pneumonia can present similarly, but there is lung eosinophilia without peripheral eosinophilia.]

31) A 34-year-old woman presented with a 6-week history of progressive weakness. She especially noticed this while brushing her hair, and it had gotten to the point that she was unable to fully complete this task due to the weakness. During the workup for this problem, a centrally located pulmonary nodule was found. This turned out to be malignant. Which of the following problems is *not* commonly associated with this cancer?

   A. SIADH.
   B. Hypercalcemia.
   C. Very aggressive.
   D. Ectopic ACTH production.
   E. Most treatment is palliative only.

[B. This patient has Eaton-Lambert syndrome caused by small cell lung cancer. Hypercalcemia is not associated with small cell cancer. It is usually seen in squamous cell cancer and, occasionally, large cell.]

32) What is the proper treatment for a pregnant patient in her first trimester for VTE prophylaxis?

   A. Low-dose SQ heparin.
   B. LMWH.
   C. Warfarin.
   D. Adjusted-dose heparin.

[B.]

33) A 45-year-old man was found to have a 1 cm solitary pulmonary nodule on chest x-ray. The nodule has "popcorn" calcifications. What is the proper treatment?

   A. Any therapy will only be palliative.
   B. Biopsy scalene lymph nodes.
   C. Just follow it with periodic chest x-rays.
   D. Bronchoscopy with biopsy and brushings.
   E. Surgery provides the only possibility of cure.

[C. Any type of calcification in a lung lesion means it is benign. "Popcorn" calcifications are seen with hamartomas. These are monitored for a period of 2 years for signs of any growth. Solitary pulmonary nodules without calcifications are also watched for 2 years in *low-risk* patients (actually, because of fear of lawsuits, they are usually worked up, but on the test you say they can be watched).]

34) In the following situations, should INH prophylaxis be started?
   A) A 25-year-old patient with no medical problems and no known exposure is found to have a 12 mm PPD. Chest x-ray is clear.
   B) A 36-year-old patient with AIDS has an 8 mm PPD.
   C) A 32-year-old nurse with no known exposure and 10 mm PPD.
   D) A nursing home patient with an 11 mm PPD.

[A. No; low-risk patients require 15 mm. B. Yes; for AIDS patients or known exposure, 5 mm is indication for prophylaxis. C. Yes. D. Yes.]

35) A 65-year-old man with history of COPD and alcoholism presents to the ER with a temperature of 101°F, cough, and confusion. Chest x-ray shows RLL patchy infiltrates. Sputum shows PMNs with no organisms. What is the best treatment?

   A. 3rd generation cephalosporin alone.
   B. 3rd generation cephalosporin plus azithromycin.
   C. PCN G.
   D. Gentamicin + 3rd-gen ceph.
   E. Erythromycin alone.

[B. Because he is 65 and has a comorbid condition of COPD and alcoholism he is at increased risk for penicillin-resistant pneumococcus as well as *Mycoplasma*, *Chlamydophilia* and enteric Gram-negative bacteria. He also has confusion, which is associated with both *Mycoplasma* and *Legionella* lung infections. Thus, of the antibiotics given, a 3rd generation cephalosporin plus azithromycin is the best treatment of choice. A 3rd generation cephalosporin alone would be appropriate if he had pneumococcus but would not get atypical organisms, and PCN G and erythromycin alone is worrisome in a patient with increased risk of resistant pneumococcus. Enteric Gram negatives in a community-acquired pneumonia are unlikely to require gentamicin therapy.]

36) A 22-year-old woman presents with sore throat, laryngitis, and cough. Rapid *Strep* is negative. Chest x-ray shows patchy infiltrates. What is the best treatment? Use the same answer options as in #35.

[E. This patient has *Chlamydophilia pneumoniae* pneumonia (TWAR). Laryngitis is the buzzword for TWAR. Otherwise, signs and symptoms are similar to *Mycoplasma pneumonia* infection. Treat TWAR with macrolides or doxycycline for 3 weeks.]

37) 55-year-old alcoholic presents to ER with a fever and coughing up bloody sputum. Chest x-ray shows bulging interlobar fissures. What is the best treatment? Use the same answer options as in #35.

[B. This is a sick man with CAP and a risk modifier (alcoholic). Even though the "bulging interlobar fissures" suggest *Klebsiella* pneumonia, the empiric treatment must cover DRSP and the atypical organisms also.]

38) A patient with a seizure disorder presents with a cavitating pneumonia. On physical exam, he has putrid breath and decayed teeth. Sputum Gram stain shows high WBC count and multiple organisms. What is the best treatment?

A. 3rd generation cephalosporin for 10 days.
B. Erythromycin for 3 weeks.
C. Fluoroquinolones for 7–10 days.
D. Gentamicin and 3rd gen ceph for 10 days.
E. Clindamycin.

[E. Aspiration pneumonia is common in seizure patients.]

39) A 33-year-old patient presents with a 2-week history of a cough only, occasionally productive with slight mucoid sputum. With onset of symptoms, the patient had a sore throat and headache. Chest x-ray shows patchy infiltrates. What is the most specific test to confirm the etiology of his pneumonia?

A. Quellung reaction.
B. KOH smear.
C. Cold agglutinins.
D. Counter-immune electrophoresis (CIE).
E. Specific IgM antibody.
F. Direct immunofluorescent antigen (DIF).

[E. This patient probably has *Mycoplasma* pneumonia. Titers > 1:64 are positive. Cold agglutinins are nonspecific IgM antibodies, which are positive only 50% of the time and are found in other diseases.]

40) A 55-year-old man presents with a 4–5 year history of progressive dyspnea. Physical exam reveals clubbing, dry inspiratory rales, and inspirations longer than exhalations. Which of the following is not true?

A. Pulmonary hypertension may develop.
B. An elevated angiotensin-converting enzyme level is likely.
C. May be associated with a high ESR.
D. Open lung biopsy is usually required for diagnosis.
E. PFTs show progressive restriction

[B. This patient has idiopathic pulmonary fibrosis. An elevated angiotensin-converting enzyme level is a nonspecific finding, usually thought of occurring in sarcoidosis; but it may also be elevated in berylliosis, TB, and leprosy, among other diseases.]

OPEN-ENDED QUESTIONS

41) Name the 5 causes of hypoxemia. Which type will respond the least to 100% O_2?

[V/Q mismatch, R-to-L shunting, hypoventilation, decreased diffusion, and high altitude (low F_iO_2). R-to-L shunting.]

42) If a patient with a pulmonary embolus has a normal O_2, would you expect the PCO_2 to be normal, high, or low?

[Low.]

43) On the hemoglobin O_2 saturation chart, what factors will shift the graph to the right, and what does this shift mean?

[Increased temp, acidosis, increased phosphate; decreased affinity for O_2.]

44) What is the difference between a lung capacity and a lung volume?

[There are 4 basic functional volumes of which the lung is made. A "capacity" is equal to ≥ 2 of these basic volumes.]

45) In what lung disease can the FEV_1/FVC be higher than normal? Is the total lung capacity increased or decreased in this disease?

[Restrictive lung disease; decreased.]

46) What types of salicylates may an aspirin-sensitive asthma patient be safely given?

[Sodium and choline salicylates.]

47) What is the most common test used to confirm the diagnosis of asthma? What principle is this test based on?

[Methacholine challenge. Nonspecific hyperirritability.]

48) What is the first choice of bronchodilators used in the rescue treatment of acute asthma?

[Beta-agonists.]

49) Name 6 factors that increase the clearance of theophylline.

[Charcoal-broiled meat, Rifampin, Adolescence, Phenobarbital and Phenytoin, Smoking (CRAPS).]

50) Theophylline increases the clearance of (name at least 2 drugs):

[Lithium and phenytoin.]

51) What is the minimum goal for the treatment of acute asthma as reflected by the blood gases?

[A room air P_aO_2 of at least 60 mm Hg or O_2 sat of 90% is the usual goal. This is also the goal for supplemental oxygen before other treatment is initiated.]

52) What type of emphysema (centroacinar or panacinar) is seen in smokers, and what type is seen in alpha-1 antitrypsin deficiency?

[Smokers: centroacinar; alpha-1: panacinar.]

53) In emphysema, the TLC is increased, so why is the vital capacity decreased?

[Even greater increase in residual volume.]

54) COPD patients are often treated with O_2 and exercise. Which improves symptoms and which will prolong life?

[Both improve symptoms; only O_2 prolongs life.]

55) State the criteria for starting chronic O_2 in a COPD patient.

[Chronic P_aO_2 of < 55 or < 59 with evidence of cor pulmonale or erythrocytosis.]

56) How many hours per day should chronic O_2 be used in the above patient?

[24 hr/day is best. For other patients, the hours per day are dependent on the circumstances that cause the low $S_{P_aO_2}$—if only with exercise, only needs while exerting +/- sleeping.]

57) What is the most common disease state associated with bronchiectasis? How is bronchiectasis best diagnosed?

[Cystic fibrosis. High-resolution CT or helical/spiral CT.]

58) In bronchiectasis, will chronic antibiotic prophylaxis prevent progression of the disease?

[No.]

59) How is hypersensitivity pneumonitis different from eosinophilic pneumonia?

[Eosinophilic pneumonia, in the acute form, has eosinophils in the infiltrates, blood, and sputum. No eosinophils are found in hypersensitivity pneumonitis.]

60) How do pleural thickening and pleural plaques differ from actual asbestosis?

[Pleural plaques occur in mid-thorax and are benign; asbestosis is parenchymal fibrosis occurring in the bases and is associated with lung cancer.]

61) What dose of beryllium is required to cause berylliosis? In what way is berylliosis similar to sarcoidosis? How is berylliosis diagnosed and treated?

[Very small doses will cause it. Both cause hilar lymphadenopathy. Diagnose with the beryllium lymphocyte transformation test. Treat with corticosteroids.]

62) In idiopathic pulmonary fibrosis (IPF), what is the best test for determining improvement in disease activity?

[Change in A-a O_2 difference response to exercise.]

63) In which of the collagen vascular diseases do you expect to find necrobiotic nodules in the upper lung zones?

[RA.]

64) In which of the connective tissue diseases is there always pulmonary (but *not* pleural) involvement?

[Scleroderma.]

65) In which of the connective tissue diseases is there pulmonary hypertension out of proportion to the pulmonary disease or chest x-ray changes?

[Scleroderma.]

66) How can you differentiate between cryptogenic organizing pneumonia and IPF?

[IPF is more insidious in onset (> 6 mo for IPF vs. 1–2 mo for COP) and patients do not have fever.]

67) How are serum angiotensin-converting enzyme levels (SACE) used in the diagnosis of sarcoidosis?

[They are nonspecific and considered of *no* use.]

68) What are the indications for corticosteroids in sarcoidosis, and in what way do corticosteroids affect disease progression?

[Corticosteroids have *not* been proven to induce remissions in sarcoidosis, although they do decrease the symptoms and PFTs improve. Inhaled corticosteroids decrease the respiratory symptoms and may be used instead of systemic corticosteroids if the disease is mainly in the lungs. Indications for *systemic* corticosteroids are involvement of other organs (eyes, heart, CNS), severe pulmonary symptoms, severe skin lesions, and persistent hypercalcemia.]

69) What type of diabetes has eosinophilic granuloma (Langerhans cell granulomatosis or eosinophilic granulomatosis) been known to cause?

[Diabetes insipidus.]

70) What type of ILD can cause a chylous pleural effusion?

[Lymphangioleiomyomatosis (RA causes a pseudochylous effusion).]

71) What disease do you expect in a patient with a purulent nasal discharge, epistaxis, and RBCs in the urine, but without pulmonary symptoms?

[Wegener granulomatosis.]

72) Which of the vasculitides causing ILD may progress to histiocytic lymphoma?

[*Lymphoma*toid granulomatosis.]

73) Which of the granulomatoses causing ILD is associated with asthma and eosinophilia? Name 2 other non-granulomatous causes of ILD that are associated with asthma and peripheral eosinophilia.

[Allergic granulomatosis of Churg-Strauss. Eosinophilic pneumonia and ABPA.]

74) Can a male patient with chronic sinusitis and clubbing have cystic fibrosis if none of his children have sinusitis and clubbing?

[No. Males with CF are sterile!]

75) What are the ECG and chest x-ray findings with primary and secondary pulmonary hypertension?

[EKG: right axis deviation. CXR: engorged pulmonary arteries; RV hypertrophy.]

76) What are common causes of secondary pulmonary hypertension outside of the U.S.?

[Filariasis and schistosomiasis and mitral valve disease.]

77) What are the initial tests done in the workup of a pleural effusion? If an exudative effusion is found, what other tests are necessary for the workup?

[Appearance, pleural fluid protein and LDH, and serum protein and LDH. If the effusion is transudative, no other tests are needed. If exudative, do cell count with diff, cytology, Gram stain and C+S, glucose, and amylase.]

78) Name the protein ratio, LDH, and LDH ratio that differentiate between transudative and exudative pleural effusions.

[Transudative: protein ratio (effusion-to-serum) < 0.5, LDH < 200, and LDH ratio < 0.6. Exudative effusion specimens have values all greater than the above.]

79) If the protein ratio is < 0.5, and the LDH ratio is > 0.6, what disease requires consideration?

[Cancer.]

80) What are the triglyceride levels that define chylous and pseudochylous pleural effusions?

[Chylous: > 115 mg/dl; pseudochylous: < 50.]

81) Do chylous or pseudochylous pleural effusion specimens clear with centrifugation?

[No, neither the chylous nor pseudochylous specimens clear with centrifugation.]

82) Name the possible diagnoses for the following pleural fluid glucose levels: 80, 60, and 20.

[80: TB; 60: cancer or empyema; 20: RA.]

83) If pleural fluid ANA is positive, what 2 tests are now done, and why?

[anti-ds DNA and antihistone; both SLE and drug-induced lupus cause an ANA+ pleural fluid.]

84) After a thoracentesis, does intrathoracic volume typically increase or decrease?

[Decrease!]

85) How do the presentations of atypical pneumonias differ from those of bacterial pneumonias?

[Atypical pneumonias are more likely to have an insidious onset with a predominance of constitutional symptoms, nonproductive cough, and normal or slightly high WBCs on CBC whereas bacterial pneumonias are more likely to have an abrupt onset with high fever and a CBC with a high WBC with left shift.]

86) What causes of pneumonia are classically associated with the following: nursing home patient; immunoglobulin deficiency; COPD; exposure to cattle or sheep; bird farmer; hunter; explorers of bat caves; recent travel to California or Arizona; homosexual?

[Nursing home: *Klebsiella*; COPD or Ig deficiency: *Moraxella catarrhalis* and *H. influenzae*; cattle or sheep: Q fever; bird farmers: psittacosis; hunters: tularemic pneumonia; bat caves: histoplasmosis; travel to California or Arizona: Coccidioidomycosis; homosexual: PCP.]

87) What is the most common cause of community-acquired bacterial pneumonia?

[*Streptococcus pneumoniae.*]

88) How do you differentiate between a good and bad sputum sample when working up pneumonia?

[Good sputum has > 25 WBCs and < 10 epithelial cells per low power field.]

89) Name the 6 chronic problems that predispose to pneumococcal pneumonia and, therefore, are indications for the pneumococcal vaccine.

[1) Renal failure, 2) Immunosuppression, 3) Chronic heart and/or lung diseases, 4) Diabetes, 5) Multiple myeloma, 6) Alcohol abuse.]

90) What are the 2 conditions that predispose patients to *Staph aureus* pneumonia?

[1) Preceding influenza infection 2) Recent use of antibiotics not effective against *S. aureus.*]

91) In which type of pneumonia does the chest x-ray classically appear worse than the symptoms suggest?

[*Mycoplasma* pneumonia.]

92) How do you diagnose *Mycoplasma* pneumonia?

[IgM antibody by means of complement fixation]

93) Which atypical pneumonia commonly has a biphasic pattern, in which there is a sore throat initially and, 2–3 weeks later, pneumonia develops?

[*Chlamydophila pneumoniae* pneumonia.]

94) In what way does clinical suspicion affect the reading of a tuberculin skin test?

[5 mm is positive if clinical suspicion is high (close contact with documented case, positive chest x-ray, HIV);
15 mm is positive if clinical suspicion is low;
10 mm for intermediate suspicion (nursing home, jailed, drug abuser, homeless, from endemic area, exposed health care worker, certain medical conditions).]

95) If a patient has a newly positive TB skin test and no indication of reactivation tuberculosis, what treatment is done and how does it vary with the patient's age?

[INH prophylaxis no matter what the age!]

96) Outline the treatment for tuberculosis.

[INH, rifampin, pyrazinamide (PZA), and either ethambutol or streptomycin for 2 months, then continue INH and rifampin for 4 more months. See the text for much more on this.]

97) If patients do receive INH prophylaxis for TB, how are the age groups > and < 35 years old monitored differently?

[No difference. Only check enzymes if the patient has symptoms.]

98) Name 3 patient groups in which *Mycobacterium kansasii* infections may be found.

[Smokers, or patients with DM or silicosis.]

99) What is the initial drug of choice for a community-acquired pneumonia in a patient with no risk factors?

[Azithromycin, clarithromycin, or doxycycline.]

100) What tests are used to diagnose the following causes of pneumonia: *Mycoplasma, Legionella, Blastomyces, Coccidioides*?

[*Mycoplasma*: complement fixation (IgM); *Legionella*: sputum culture on special media and urinary antigen assay; *Blastomyces* and *Coccidioides*: KOH smear. Also can use immunodiffusion for *Coccidioides.*]

101) What organism is the direct immunofluorescent antigen (DIF) test used to detect?

[*Legionella*, influenza A & B, RSV, and adenovirus.]

102) How is CMV pneumonitis diagnosed? What are its related problems?

[Think of CMV if there is a mixed bag of "-itises." Patients often get concurrent pneumonitis, hepatitis (usually mild), and adrenalitis causing adrenal insufficiency! The diagnosis is confirmed if inclusion bodies are seen in samples from BAL/lung biopsy.]

103) In an AIDS patient with suspected PCP, if the sputum is negative, what is the next test done? How is PCP treated?

[Bronchoalveolar lavage (BAL); TMP/SMX or pentamidine is effective against PCP pneumonia; try TMP/SMX first, because it can eventually be given orally. Only 1/2 of PCP patients improve on the initial course of therapy (usually 3 weeks) and 1/2 get intolerable side effects from either medication. Don't forget to also give corticosteroids if the patient is hypoxic.]

104) What is the order of frequency of lung diseases in AIDS patients?

[PCP > TB/MA-I > Bacterial > CMV/HSV > Fungal.]

105) What type of lung reaction, cytotoxic or non-cytotoxic, does methotrexate cause? Bleomycin?

[Methotrexate: noncytotoxic. Bleomycin: cytotoxic.]

106) Name 3 factors that will exacerbate bleomycin lung toxicity.

[Uremia, supplemental O_2, and radiation therapy.]

107) In patients with AML, besides the normal infections, what should be considered when there are a pulmonary infiltrates?

[Hemorrhage due to infiltrates.]

108) In what type of leukemia are leukemic pulmonary infiltrates most commonly seen?

[ALL (acute lymphoblastic leukemia); leukemic infiltrate implies a high number of blasts.]

109) How long does it usually take a radiation lung reaction to present?

[Within 6 months of radiation therapy; radiation pneumonitis occurs within 6 weeks.]

110) What are the mediators released by monocytes that may help maintain the septic state?

[Tumor Necrosis Factor (TNF) and Interleukin-1.]

111) What is the most common cause of death within the first 3 days after onset of ARDS? After 3 days?

[< 3 days: the underlying problem that caused ARDS; > 3 days: sepsis.]

112) How do you diagnose pneumonia in a patient with ARDS?

[Infiltrates and leukocytosis are common in both. BAL > 10^4 or protected brush samples growing > 10^3 organisms/ml are currently the best ways to diagnose pneumonia in ARDS.]

113) Name 5 common causes of failure to wean from a ventilator.

[(DESAT): 1) Drugs (sedatives...), 2) Endotracheal tube has too small a bore, 3) Secretions, 4) Alkalemia (decreases respiratory drive), 5) Too high a P_aO_2 and too low a PCO_2 just before extubating (should keep it near the patient's baseline).]

114) If the PAWP waveform varies during respiratory cycle, how is a more accurate pulmonary artery wedge pressure determined?

[The reading should be taken at end-exhalation.]

115) In a critically ill patient, why should phosphorus level be checked?

[Hypophosphatemia decreases diaphragmatic contractility in addition to shifting the O_2 saturation curve to the left.]

116) If the patient is unable to eat after surgery, when should enteral feedings or TPN be started?

[The enteral route is used whenever possible. If the patient is unable to eat, enteral feedings or TPN should be started ASAP after the initial insult. Even though enteral feeding increases the possibility of aspiration, it is preferred over TPN, because it tends to maintain the intestinal epithelium and its natural defenses against bacteria.]

117) Are pleurisy and friction rubs seen more often with massive PEs or smaller ones? What 3 findings are more specific for massive PE?

[Pleurisy and friction rubs are actually seen more often in submassive PEs—because they are due to a distal impaction of the vessel, and so occur nearer to the pleura. There are 3 findings more specific for a massive PE: increased P2 (pulmonic heart sound), S3 and/or S4 gallop, and cyanosis.]

118) What is the only specific ECG finding occasionally seen with acute pulmonary embolus?

[The only specific (but not sensitive) heart/ECG changes seen with PE include tachycardia and right ventricle strain (i.e., acute cor pulmonale) on ECG (S_1-Q_3-T_3).]

119) If P_aO_2 and chest x-ray are not very sensitive indicators of pulmonary embolus, why are they always done in a suspected case?

[P_aO_2: To determine if the patient is hypoxemic and needs oxygen—a normal P_aO_2 has fairly good negative predictive value. Also the A-a O_2 diff can be determined from the ABGs; chest x-ray: Rule out other causes of the symptoms such as pneumonia or pneumothorax.]

120) What is the anticoagulant treatment for pulmonary embolus, where are the PTT or INR levels maintained, and how long is treatment continued?

[Unfractionated heparin (UH) is the initial treatment. It is adjusted to keep the PTT at least 1.5 x control and is given for 7–10 days. Then anticoagulant treatment is continued for 3–6 months with LMWH or with warfarin to an INR of 2.0–3.0.]

121) Why should platelet count be monitored when a patient is on heparin?

[Thrombocytopenia occasionally develops.]

122) Give the indications for using thrombolytics with acute pulmonary embolism.

[Thrombolytics now are used to treat a significant acute PE with unstable hemodynamics or decompensation. Also may be used when there is RV overload, strain, or dysfunction due to PE.]

123) When should a venacaval filter be used?

[When a patient has had a pulmonary embolus and will die if another one occurs (e.g., massive PE after either a massive MI or heart surgery). Also when there are recurring VTEs with adequate anticoagulation or when there are recurring VTEs and anticoagulant treatment is contraindicated]

124) List which patients are at highest risk, moderate risk, and lower risk for developing a pulmonary embolus.

[Patients at highest risk for a PE have an acute fracture of, or orthopedic procedure on, a lower extremity or are post-extensive pelvic/abdominal surgery for cancer. Moderate risk: any other surgery—especially in patients > 40 years old, or with CHF or pneumonia. Lower, but still significant, risk includes all immobilized patients.]

125) What is the most common type of sleep apnea and how does it present? What symptoms does the patient have?

[Obstructive. The patient has transient complete obstruction of the upper airway despite increased respiratory effort. This is followed by a loud snore.]

126) How is sleep apnea diagnosed?

[Polysomnography showing ~ ≥ 10 apneic episodes per hour while sleeping. It can be confirmed by finding oxygen desaturations > 4% with the apneic episodes.]

127) How does the risk of lung cancer decrease after quitting smoking? How does lung function improve after quitting smoking?

[The risk decreases for 15 years after smoking is stopped, until it returns to normal. Lung function also improves after smoking cessation, but not to normal.]

128) Malignant mesothelioma is usually considered pathognomonic for exposure to what material?

[Asbestos.]

129) Name the 4 major categories of lung cancer and state their relative frequency.

[Adenocarcinoma (1/3), squamous cell (1/3), small cell (1/4), and large cell (1/5)—these are rounded up (so they don't add up to exactly 100%).]

130) Which 2 lung cancers are usually central lesions and which 2 are usually peripheral lesions?

[Central: squamous and small cell (S-S-SENTRAL). Peripheral: adeno and large cell.]

131) Which lung cancer is most likely to cavitate?

[Squamous cell.]

132) What percent of solitary pulmonary nodules are malignant?

[35%!]

133) When a patient has a popcorn calcification of a solitary pulmonary nodule, what lesion does this suggest?

[A benign hamartoma. Calcified lung nodules are virtually always benign.]

134) What do all possibly curative treatments of lung cancer include?

[Surgery.]

135) What must the pre-pneumonectomy FEV_1 be to insure adequate post-op pulmonary function? If the FEV_1 is too low, what further testing should be done?

[Pre-op FEV should be > 2 liters to ensure adequate pulmonary function if a pneumonectomy is done (need a FEV_1 > 0.8 L after surgery to survive). If the FEV_1 is < 1.6 liters, do a quantitative V/Q scan to better evaluate. Resting hypercapnia usually means the patient is not a surgical candidate.]

136) What is the usual cause of superior vena caval syndrome?

[75–85% are due to bronchogenic carcinoma—usually small cell, then large cell.]

MedStudy®

12th Edition

Internal Medicine Review Core Curriculum

Nephrology

Authored by Robert A. Hannaman, MD

Many thanks to

> N. Kevin Krane, MD
> Professor of Medicine
> Chief, Clinical Nephrology
> Tulane University Health Sciences Center
> New Orleans, Louisiana

Nephrology Advisor

Table of Contents

Nephrology

Urinalysis (UA)—When there are no red blood cells (RBCs) on microscopic analysis but the urine dipstick is positive, think of hemoglobinuria or myoglobinuria.

- One unusual cause of hemoglobinuria is lysis of RBCs in a very dilute urine. RBC casts or "dysmorphic" RBCs indicate probable glomerulonephritis.
- With eosinophiluria, think of drug-induced interstitial nephritis.
- Proteinuria is the best indicator of underlying renal pathology. Normal 24-hour urine protein is < 150 mg. Greater than 2.5–3.5 gm/d (or 40–50 mg/kg/d) means significant glomerular pathology. Patients with proteinuria < 1 gm/d are more likely to have interstitial renal disease. Medullary cystic disease and obstructive uropathy are the only exceptions in which there can be pathology and a normal urine sediment with minimal proteinuria. Myeloma often results in light chain production (Bence-Jones proteinuria), which is not picked up on urine dipstick; order 24-hr urine for immunoelectrophoresis.
- Transient proteinuria is common in people during a febrile illness, after strenuous exercise, and in patients with CHF and COPD. Recheck urine when the acute situation has passed. If the repeat urinalysis is negative, the condition can be considered benign. There is an entity called benign orthostatic proteinuria, in which the proteinuria reverts to near-normal values when the patient is supine.
- Protein:Creatinine Ratio (aka the "renal ratio") is a simpler method to determine proteinuria, because it requires only a "spot" urine sample for these 2 values. The ratio of the protein:creatinine equates to the amount of protein in a 24-hour urine in gm; i.e., a protein:creatinine ratio of 3.5 = a 24-hour urine of 3.5 gm. This test has become the recommended test to determine and follow proteinuria in patients with renal disease.
- Micro-albuminuria is the earliest indication of diabetic nephropathy. It is when the amount of protein being spilled is too small an amount to be picked up on the urine dipstick. Later, in diabetic nephropathy, heavy proteinuria (nephrotic syndrome) occurs. Micro-albuminuria also may be an indicator of early glomerular injury in diseases other than diabetes, including hypertension—in which case it is a risk factor for cardiovascular disease. Causes of false-positive urine albumin on dipstick include a very alkaline urine with a pH > 8, fever, CHF, UTI, and a very concentrated urine.

Serum creatinine is the common screening measure of renal function; however, this value can vary depending on the amount produced. Creatinine is produced by muscle tissue and the more muscle tissue one has, the higher the value. Also, if muscle tissue breaks down (rhabdomyolysis), creatinine values can rise acutely. Cooked meat converts creatine in the muscle to creatinine which, when eaten, is absorbed and enters the creatinine pool. With aging, there is less muscle mass, and the creatinine does not rise despite reduced renal function.

Serum creatinine is increased by: cimetidine, probenecid, and trimethoprim (consider this if there is increased creatinine in an AIDS patient treated with TMP/SMX for PCP). These drugs decrease the tubular secretion of creatinine. Acetone and cefoxitin interfere with the test for creatinine, and may give falsely elevated results. An elevated (> 20:1) BUN/Cr ratio indicates either prerenal azotemia (low flow and increased absorption) or increased protein breakdown. The increased protein breakdown can be due to increased protein intake, GI bleed, TPN, catabolic states, or steroids that increase protein turnover.

Glomerular filtration rate (GFR) is the most accurate way to measure renal function. Traditionally, this has been calculated as the Creatinine Clearance (CrCl), in ml/min = UV/P, where UV is the total urine creatine/24 hours divided by the serum creatinine (sCR). The easiest and most accurate method to calculate GFR is to download the MDRD formula, which uses only serum values and accounts for race, sex, and nutritional status. The Cockcroft-Gault formula is another acceptable way to determine GFR as CrCl:

$$CrCl = \left(140 - age_{years}\right) \times \left(\frac{Weight}{72 \times sCR}\right)$$

$$CrCl = mg/min$$
$$age = years$$
$$weight = kg$$
$$sCR = mg/dL$$

(CrCl x .85 = CrCl for women)

As mentioned, the creatinine clearance may be affected by certain drugs (probenecid, cimetidine, trimethoprim), which decrease the secretion of creatinine, and thereby cause a decreased creatinine clearance—with no change in GFR. Another time the creatinine clearance does not reflect GFR is in advanced renal disease, when secretion is increased by the tubules. In this case, measured creatinine clearance is higher than actual GFR.

The fractional excretion of sodium (FE_{Na}) is a measurement of Na^+ excreted over the total filtered load of Na^+. It is most useful in evaluating acute renal failure and is primarily used to differentiate prerenal azotemia from acute tubular necrosis (ATN). It is typically < 1% in prerenal azotemia and > 2% in ATN. Contrast-induced ATN is an exception, where the FE_{Na} can be < 1%.

$$FE_{Na}(\%) = \frac{\frac{uNa}{sNa}}{\frac{uCr}{sCr}} \times 100 = \left(\frac{uNa \times sCr}{sNa \times uCr}\right) \times 100$$

Use renal biopsy to diagnose unexplained causes of acute renal failure, nephrotic syndrome, and glomerulonephritis. In transplant patients, it assists in distinguishing between cyclosporine or tacrolimus toxicity, ATN, viral infections, and rejection episodes.

-emia vs. -osis—If the pH is < 7.4, the patient has acidemia; if > 7.4, the patient has alkalemia. Either one of these states may include various combinations of metabolic/respiratory acidosis or alkalosis.

Remember, significant alkalemia of any etiology can cause the diffuse paresthesias/numbness and muscle spasms we usually

notes

Table 4-1: Rules of Thumb for Acid-Base Problems

EQUILIBRIUM REACTIONS BETWEEN P_aCO_2 AND HCO_3^-		Then pH changes: (Acute/Chronic)	Then HCO_3^- changes: (Acute/Chronic)	Then P_aCO_2 changes:
RESPIRATORY DISORDERS	If P_aCO_2 decreases by 10	.08/.04	-2/-5	
	If P_aCO_2 increases by 10	-.08/-.04	1/4	
METABOLIC DISORDERS	If HCO_3^- decreases by 10			-12
	If HCO_3^- increases by 10			6

associate with acute hyperventilation; the high pH increases the fraction of bound calcium. The resulting decrease in ionized calcium produces these symptoms of hypocalcemia (serum calcium = ionized + bound = no change)! This also can be induced by rapid overload with intravenous HCO_3^- or citrate, such as after massive blood transfusion.

ACID-BASE DISORDERS
MECHANISMS

There is really only one chemical equation you must know to calculate and understand all acid-base problems. This is the Henderson equation. It is derived from the bicarbonate buffer equation:

$$HCO_3^- + H^+ \leftrightarrow H_2CO_3 \leftrightarrow H_2O + CO_2 \qquad \text{(eq 1)}$$

H_2CO_3 is carbonic acid. HCO_3^- is bicarbonate. CO_2 is carbon dioxide. These 3 molecules are in equilibrium with one another. From the above equation is derived the "beloved" Henderson-Hasselbalch equation. (Derivation shown in appendix A at the end of the Nephrology section).

$$pH = pK + \log(HCO_3^-/.03 P_aCO_2) \qquad \text{(eq 2)}$$

which can be more easily used as:

$$H^+ = 24(P_aCO_2 / HCO_3^-) \qquad \text{(eq 3)}$$

This equation reflects the facts that the serum pH is made up of respiratory (P_aCO_2) and metabolic (HCO_3^-) components, and that it is the ratio of these values in the blood that determines pH and not their absolute level. The kidney regulates the HCO_3^- while the lungs regulate the P_aCO_2.

Several important concepts determine acid-base status. These include [Know]:
1) What effect ventilation, which is reflected in the P_aCO_2, has on pH and HCO_3^-.
2) What effect metabolic alkalosis or acidosis, reflected in the HCO_3^-, has on P_aCO_2 (ventilation).
3) Anion Gap and Osmolal Gap.
4) Whether disturbances are simple (only 1 abnormality) vs. mixed acid-base disturbances.

As for 1 and 2: Table 4-1 gives some rough rules of thumb (in practice, a nomogram is generally used). Know that the body's ventilatory response to metabolic acid-base changes is immediately reflected in the P_aCO_2: Respiratory rate increases (with resulting decrease in P_aCO_2) in response to metabolic acidosis. Similarly, respiratory rate decreases (with a resulting increase of P_aCO_2) in response to metabolic alkalosis.

On the other hand, it takes much longer for the kidneys to compensate for sustained changes in acid-base status. This is why the table shows both acute and chronic changes in pH and HCO_3^-. Examples soon follow that help clarify the table. But first, we'll discuss anion gap, osmolal gap, and causes of acid-base abnormalities.

ANION GAP

The normal serum anion gap is 12. $AG = Na^+ - (HCO_3^- + Cl^-)$. See Table 4-2 regarding its derivation, and refer to Table 4-3 as you go through the following discussion. Use the anion gap in the diagnostic workup of metabolic acidosis.

Urine anion gap (UAG) is useful when working up a normal anion gap acidosis (see next). $UAG = Na^+ + K^+ - Cl^-$, which are the major ions in the urine. The Normal is -10 to $+10$.

Table 4-2: Derivation of the Anion Gap

Anion Gap derivation (NO need to memorize!)

Because the H^+ may be produced by any acid, we can say:

$HCO_3^- + (H^+ + A^-)$ is in equilibrium with $H_2O + CO_2 + A^-$

The anions in blood include HCO_3^-, Cl^-, phosphate (phos), sulfate, albumin, and organic acids. The cations are Na^+, K^+, Ca^{++}, and Mg^{++}. Because plasma remains neutral, the true anion gap (AG) is zero or:

$(Na^+ + K^+ + Ca^{++} + Mg^{++}) - (HCO_3^- + Cl^- + phos + sulfate + albumin + organic acids) = 0$

This is very cumbersome so some normally unmeasured ions have been dropped and it has been reduced to the major ions and is:

$AG = Na^+ - (Cl^- + HCO_3^-)$.

Fiddling with the equation shows the AG is actually a measurement of the (unmeasured anions) - (unmeasured cations):

$AG = Na^+ - (Cl^- + HCO_3^-) = (phos+sulfate+albumin+organic acids) - (K^+ + Ca^{++} + Mg^{++})$

This is usually about 24 meq/l - 12 meq/l = 12 meq/l. Because the cations' concentration rarely changes much, it is easiest to just think of the AG as a measurement of the unmeasured anions. Indeed, it is usually taught this way.

notes ✓ Even in chr. resp. acidosis, the serum HCO_3^- does NOT inc above 38 meq/L

✓ If $P_{CO_2} > 55$, usually suggests an additional 1° resp. acidosis.

✓ For resp. alkalosis alone, HCO_3^- NEVER falls below 12 meq/L. (response to)

✓ meta. alkalosis ⟨ saline responsive — here the urine chloride <10 / saline resistant

Calculated osmolal gap: $2 \times Na^+ + \frac{Glucose}{18} + \frac{BUN}{2-8}$

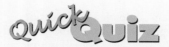

In this text, "anion gap" will refer to "serum anion gap," and "urine anion gap" (UAG) will always be mentioned as such.

METABOLIC ACIDOSIS

Metabolic acidosis occurs with:
1) overproduction of lactic or ketoacids,
2) HCO_3^- wasting (renal tubular acidosis or diarrhea),
3) under-excretion of acid (renal failure),
4) poisonings by agents that are metabolized to acids.

Normal Anion Gap Acidosis

Normal anion gap (NAG) acidosis (or "hyperchloremic" acidosis) accompanies commensurate increase of Cl^- and decrease of HCO_3^-. NAG acidosis occurs from:
• a loss of HCO_3^- (GI or renal [as in RTA—pg 4-9]),
• inability of the kidney to excrete endogenous acids, or
• ingestion of organic acids (NH^4).

With HCO_3^- loss, Cl^- is retained to maintain electrical neutrality, and so serum Cl^- level increases. It is hard to distinguish renal tubular acidosis (RTA) from GI loss of HCO_3^-, so the Urine Anion Gap (UAG) is used, because it directly reflects the kidney's excretion of NH_4^+.

You see UAG > 10 in renal normal anion gap metabolic acidosis (RTA).

You see UAG < -10 in extrarenal (i.e., probably GI) normal anion gap metabolic acidosis. More on RTA on pg 4-9.

High Anion Gap Acidosis

High anion gap acidoses are more interesting. On the electrolytes panel, the only abnormality is a low HCO_3^-—i.e., there is no equivalent increase in Cl^-. Because the net charge is always neutral, there must be an increase in the unmeasured anions. The most common causes are ketoacidosis (diabetic, alcoholic, and starvation), lactic acidosis, (including D-lactic acidosis), uremia, and toxins (salicylates, ethylene glycol [makes glycolic and oxalic acid], toluene, and methanol [makes formic acid]).

Alcoholic ketoacidosis responds well to dextrose solutions. In ketoacidosis, there is classically volume depletion, a normal Cl^-, and a high anion gap...but 1/2 of diabetics with DKA present without volume depletion, and these tend to have a high Cl^- with a normal anion gap!

D-lactic acidosis occurs in patients with short bowels who present with obtundation. Responds to dextrose fluids.

Patients who drink methanol produce formaldehyde and formic acid, resulting in a high anion gap acidosis.

Ethylene glycol (antifreeze) forms glycolic acid and oxalic acid, resulting in a high anion gap acidosis and calcium oxalate crystals in the urine.

Patients drinking isopropyl alcohol can have significant ketosis without acidosis, because isopropyl alcohol breaks down to acetone. So suspect this if the patient arrives stuporous with a fruity smell on his breath and has normal chemistry except high ketones.

3 tests should immediately be performed in a patient with an unexplained high AG acidosis:
• urine + serum ketone levels,
• lactic acid level, and the
• osmolal gap.

The osmolal gap is the difference between measured and calculated osmolality. Calculated osmolality is:

$$Osm_{calc} = 2[Na] + BUN/2.8 + glucose/18$$
$$\text{Normal osmolal gap is} < 10.$$

A large osmolal gap (usually > 20) in an intoxicated patient with a high AG acidosis should lead to the immediate consideration of poisoning by one of the alcohols (ethanol, ethylene glycol, or methanol). Conditions that cause an osmolal gap alone are covered in "Poisonings" in the General Internal Medicine section.

Table 4-3: Anion Gap vs. Causes of Metabolic Acidosis
The normal anion gap is 12.
$AG = Na^+ - (Cl^- + HCO_3^-)$
Causes of INCREASED anion gap metabolic acidosis: Severe CKD (CRF): decreased acid (especially NH_4) excretion - commonest   Ketoacidosis: diabetic, alcoholic, starvation   Lactic acidosis: drugs, toxins, circulatory compromise   Poisonings: salicylates, methanol, ethylene glycol
Causes of NORMAL anion gap metabolic acidosis: Renal tubular acidosis   Diarrhea   Carbonic anhydrase inhibitors   Hyperalimentation with TPN

notes

METABOLIC ALKALOSIS

Metabolic alkalosis usually results from volume contraction caused by diuretics or vomiting, which also causes a loss of HCl. With volume contraction the urinary Cl^- is < 10 mEq/L, because there is more avid resorption of NaCl (to maintain intravascular volume). If urinary Cl^- is > 10, think of other causes of alkalosis, such as Cushing syndrome, 1° hyperaldosteronism, severe hypokalemia, or increased intake of HCO_3^-.

Alkalosis itself can cause decreased serum K^+ from increased K^+ loss (see distal tubule, pg 4-8) and increased cellular K^+ uptake.

Treatment of severe metabolic alkalosis (> 7.55) requires KCl, NaCl, or occasionally HCl. Avoid KCl when there is renal insufficiency, and avoid NaCl in CHF. Use HCl when there is both renal insufficiency and CHF. When giving intravenous HCl, use only 0.1N solution, because the 0.3N solution can cause breakdown of the blood vessels. Even the 0.1N solution of HCl must be given via a central line. Ammonium chloride (NH_4Cl), an oral drug, is an alternative treatment that is only rarely used. A preferable drug is the carbonic anhydrase inhibitor, acetazolamide (Diamox®), which increases bicarbonate excretion.

ANALYSIS OF ACID-BASE PROBLEMS

The sequence used in analyzing acid-base status:
1) ABGs: P_aCO_2 and pH
2) Anion gap: $AG = Na^+ - (HCO_3^- + Cl^-)$
3) Osmolal gap: $Osm_{calc} = 2[Na] + BUN/2.8 + glucose/18$
4) Serum bicarb: HCO_3^-
5) Chloride: Cl^-
6) Urine anion gap (for NAG metabolic acidosis)

When analyzing acid-base status:
1) Look at the pH. Is the patient acidemic or alkalemic?
2) Is the primary problem respiratory or metabolic? Look at the P_aCO_2—which gives the status of ventilation (hyper-/hypo)—then look at the HCO_3^- to see if it reflects a metabolic abnormality.
3) Is this a simple or mixed acid-base disturbance? In simple disorders, the kidneys and lungs respond in a predictable physiologic response, for which we can use simple calculations or nomograms. For example, in respiratory alkalosis, the approximate change in pH = +.08 for each change in P_aCO_2 of -10. If the pH change is less than this, there is some compensatory metabolic acidosis. (Again, we usually use nomograms; these values are just an approximation.)

Acute respiratory acidosis is just the opposite. For each increase in P_aCO_2 of 10, the pH decreases ~ 0.08. Any change in pH less than this indicates some compensatory metabolic alkalosis. Then check the P_aO_2. Table 4-4 lists some sample ABGs with likely causes.

Clues to Mixed Disorders: Severe acidosis or alkalosis (look for combined metabolic/respiratory components) or "normal" pH with an AG (look for both acidosis and alkalosis in the same patient, like the diabetic presented a few paragraphs below).

Note: Serum bicarbonate is often represented as "CO_2." This is a misnomer and just shorthand for HCO_3^-. Also note that serum bicarbonate is measured HCO_3^-, whereas the HCO_3^- readout in the ABGs is a derived value using pH and P_aCO_2. "Measured" is more accurate than "derived." In the following discussion, I'm using measured HCO_3^-.

Where does the serum HCO_3^- enter into the picture? First remember that HCO_3^- and CO_2 are in equilibrium in the blood. Anytime P_aCO_2 changes, there should be an immediate change in HCO_3^-. This acute change is minimal, as you can see in Table 4-1, and reflects the different stresses on, and buffering by, the bicarbonate buffer system (eq 1). Because normal serum bicarbonate is 23–28 mmol/L, the acute

pH	P_aCO_2	P_aO_2	ACID-BASE STATUS*	EXAMPLES...
7.56	20	90	Acute respiratory alkalosis	Acute hyperventilation episode
7.56	20	50	Acute resp alk due to hypoxia	Acute asthma/ PE/ chest trauma
7.44	25	90	Chronic resp alk w metab compensation	CNS problem, chronic hyperventilation
7.43	30	60	As above, but w hypoxia	COPD, "Pink puffer"
7.40	40	50	Normal except hypoxia	Pt in transition to respiratory failure!
7.24	60	80	Acute resp acidosis	Sedative overdose
7.16	70	50	Acute resp acidosis w hypoxia	Resp failure from hypoxia
7.37	60	60	Resp acidosis w metabolic compensation	COPD, "Blue bloater" - CO_2 retainer
7.44	60	90	Metabolic alkalosis w resp comp	Bicarbonate overdose
7.36	28	90	Metabolic acidosis w resp comp	Sepsis, ASA overdose, renal failure...

Table 4-4: Examples of Abnormal Acid-Base Status

* assuming consistent HCO_3^- and chloride (see text).

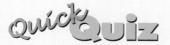

change is often not noticeable. If the change in ventilatory rate (P_aCO_2) persists, the kidneys react, and either retain or get rid of bicarbonate in order to return the serum pH to normal range. This is the cause for the larger changes in HCO_3^- with chronic changes in P_aCO_2. Note that the P_aCO_2 and HCO_3^- should always move in the same direction; e.g., chronic hypoventilation → increased P_aCO_2 → respiratory acidosis → renal retention of HCO_3^- → increased serum HCO_3^- → normalized serum pH.

If the HCO_3^- does not move in the same direction as the P_aCO_2, or not as much as it should, it means there is a third abnormality! It can get pretty strange. Example: if, in the first example of Table 4-4, you find that the HCO_3^- is 29, this indicates that it is not an acute respiratory alkalosis but rather a chronic/compensated respiratory alkalosis with an additional metabolic alkalosis.

There is one final clue useful with anion gap acidoses. The Cl is normally 2/3 of Na. It is lower in endogenous metabolic alkalosis and higher in most metabolic acidoses except high anion gap acidosis. To see how this helps, study the following example: A young patient with IDDM comes in complaining of persistent vomiting and has the following blood work: Na 135, K 3.2, Cl 75, bicarb 24. ABGs: 7.40, 40, 96. The chief resident is sending him home because the ABG values are normal. What do you think?

You glance at the values and tell your chief resident to admit the patient for DKA (especially impressive if you are an intern). What you saw was an increased anion gap "caused by" a low Cl. The low Cl suggests a metabolic alkalosis, probably from vomiting, which (because the pH is normal) must be neutralizing a high anion gap metabolic acidosis—almost certainly DKA in this case. You might see something similar in a patient with salicylate poisoning.

FLUID AND ELECTROLYTES

Normal osmolality is usually 282 ± 2 mOsm/kg H_2O. If there are none of the abnormalities previously mentioned (i.e., ethylene glycol poisoning), measured osmolality is equal to calculated osmolality:

$$Osm_{calc} = 2[Na] + Glucose/18 + BUN/2.8$$

If glucose and BUN are normal, use just 2 x [Na] to quickly see if the calculated osmolality is about normal.

ADH levels are regulated by several mechanisms. Osmoreceptors in the hypothalamus provide the primary stimulus for ADH control. Volume receptors (stretch receptors) in the left atrium, and possibly the pulmonary veins and blood vessel receptors, supply strong stimuli when activated. The strongest stimulant for ADH release is significant volume loss resulting in hypotension; e.g., hemorrhage. This stimulates both the stretch receptors and baroreceptors. Increased levels of BUN and glucose do not cause ADH secretion. ADH acts on the collecting duct to increase water permeability, thereby increasing urine concentration. More in the Endocrinology section on ADH.

Volume status of the patient with an electrolyte abnormality is critical in determining the treatment. In general, if the patient is edematous, there is volume overload. If the patient has the clinical signs of volume loss, there is, of course, a volume deficit. If there is neither of these, the patient is considered isovolemic. Remember: Assess volume by clinical standards. Signs of volume loss include (in increasing order) tachycardia, narrowing pulse pressure, orthostatic hypotension, and resting tachycardia with hypotension. Checking these should be part of the evaluation of volume status in all patients with electrolyte abnormalities.

HYPONATREMIA

Isotonic and Hypertonic

Low Na^+ is the most common electrolyte abnormality. It is further classified by osmolality as isotonic, hypertonic, or hypotonic. Remember, the first step after finding hyponatremia is determining serum osmolality and glucose.

1) Isotonic hyponatremia occurs when protein or lipids displace sodium, as in multiple myeloma (MM) and hyperlipidemia. There is an increased osmolal gap: The measured serum osmolality is normal, while the calculated osmolality is low because of the low Na^+.

2) Hypertonic: Both glucose and mannitol cause an osmotic shift of water out of cells, which dilutes plasma Na^+. Remember: For each 100 mg/dl increase in glucose, sodium concentration decreases by 1.6.

3) Hypotonic (discussed now)

Hypotonic

By far, the largest low-Na^+ subgroup is the hypotonic group. The hypotonicity causes intracellular swelling, which may result in neuromuscular excitability, seizures, and coma—usually when the Na^+ goes acutely < 120. If the sodium level decreases slowly, the cells re-equilibrate and do not swell enough to cause these symptoms. The hypotonic group is further subdivided by volume status: low–high–normal.

The serum Na^+ is a measure of body water and reflects the ratio of total body Na^+ to total body water. In the patient with hypotonic low-Na^+, the first thing to do is clinically assess patient's volume:

Hypotonic...**Low** Volume

The low-volume patients have lost both water and Na^+ but more Na^+ than water. This is caused by:
- diuretics
- GI losses (vomiting and diarrhea)
- adrenal insufficiency

In adrenal insufficiency, low aldosterone causes decreased active Na resorption. This results in Na^+ and water wasting, high K^+, and a mild metabolic acidosis.

Hypotonic...**High** Volume

The high-volume hyponatremic patients usually retain water and Na^+—but water more than Na^+—so some have normal and most (90%!) have even elevated *total body* Na^+. Often they have dependent edema and JVD. Causes include:
- Low-output CHF
- Edema-causing states (hypoalbuminemia, cirrhosis, and nephrotic syndrome)
- Acute or chronic renal failure

Normal treatment is restriction of water and Na^+. If the patient has CHF +/- pulmonary edema, add loop diuretics or ACEI/ARBs to the treatment. Avoid lithium and demeclocycline, because they might decrease GFR, causing an increased salt retention. Also avoid chronic, oral thiazide diuretics, because they impair urinary diluting ability (use only loop diuretics if needed).

Careful! It's easy to precipitate renal failure by rapidly diuresing a high-volume cirrhotic patient with decreased CrCl. You have to be especially careful with cirrhotics because they may have a normal serum creatinine, with even a low GFR. They tend to have decreased muscle mass, which means less muscle breakdown and ultimately, even with a decreased GFR, a normal serum creatinine.

Hypotonic...**Normal** Volume (SIADH)

The normal-volume patients usually have SIADH, but this can also be caused by psychogenic polydipsia (rare), and even by diuretics if there is sufficient free water replacement. In the latter case, serum K^+ is usually low. If there is no renal pathology, the only abnormality on routine tests is hyponatremia (MM and hyperlipidemia present similarly). The serum uric acid and BUN are low (dilutional). The most serious causes of SIADH are CNS disorders (including meningitis), lung disorders, and cancer (especially small cell, but also cancers of the pancreas, duodenum, and thymus). SIADH also can be caused by drugs—especially chlorpropamide, phenothiazines, cyclophosphamide, clofibrate, and vincristine. Other causes are emetic response (increases ADH), and old age (increased ADH secretion with increased age).

Check urine osmolality to differentiate between SIADH and psychogenic polydipsia. In the former, the urine is concentrated whereas in the latter, the urine is dilute. Clue: If a patient presents with hyponatremia and a low serum uric acid and BUN, it is probably SIADH. Uric acid is usually higher in the other causes. The serum uric acid and BUN are extremely useful in differentiating hyponatremia due to SIADH

vs. diuretic-induced volume depletion. Once the diagnosis of SIADH is made, the difficulty is determining the underlying etiology. History and physical exam results point to the cause in many cases. Patients who have a negative workup (usually with a total body CT scan) should be worked up again every 1–2 years, because often a malignancy eventually shows up.

Treatment of Hyponatremia

In all types of hyponatremia, if the patient is hypovolemic, give 1–2 liters of normal saline. If the symptoms of hyponatremia are severe (e.g., coma, convulsions) and the patient is not hypovolemic, treat with 3% saline along with loop diuretics.

Give enough 3% saline over 8–12 hours to increase the serum sodium by 10 mEq/L. Calculate the mEq of Na^+ needed by multiplying total body water (60% of body weight—i.e., 60 L in a 100 kg person) x 10 mEq/L. In this case, 60 L x 10 mEq/L = 600 mEq. Each liter of 3% saline has 512 mEq of Na^+, so give ~ 1 liter over 12 hours.

Never, never give hypertonic saline rapidly (see below)! If treatment includes hypertonic saline, the rate of correction should not exceed 1–2 mmol/hr. Then switch to the treatment consistent with the etiology of the hyponatremia. If the patient is hypovolemic (e.g., diarrhea), give normal saline. If the patient has normal or high volume, place on fluid restriction. SIADH is treated with fluid restriction, and up to 900 mg/day of demeclocycline may be useful in certain refractory SIADH cases. Demeclocycline inhibits ADH stimulation of adenylate cyclase in the renal tubule. Occasionally, some use lithium carbonate (it decreases the concentrating ability of the kidney).

Demeclocycline has some interesting and important side effects. It may cause a photosensitive skin rash. It is bound to albumin, and the free drug may be nephrotoxic so, in hypoalbuminemic patients (i.e., cirrhosis or nephrotic syndrome), use a decreased dosage and carefully follow renal function.

Osmotic demyelination syndrome = Central pontine myelinolysis (because it is most prominent in the pons). It is very important not to replenish the Na^+ too quickly. In the patient with chronic severe hyponatremia, the cells that are initially enlarged due to the extracellular hypoosmolality re-equilibrate by pumping out solutes and becoming equally hypoosmotic. If the sodium concentration is raised too rapidly, the cells shrink, causing the demyelination syndrome/central pontine myelinolysis. As this implies, the chance of this occurring is much higher in patients with chronic hyponatremia who are corrected rapidly. Again: Do not treat hyponatremia with hypertonic solution unless it is severe and the patient is symptomatic. If it is treated with hypertonic saline, the rate of correction should not exceed 1–2 mmol/hr.

Cellular swelling can occur from too rapid a correction of any severe hyperosmolar state, such as hypernatremia, nonketotic hyperglycemic coma, and severe uremia (these are just the variables in the osmolality equation). Cellular swelling can cause cerebral edema, seizures, and coma.

notes

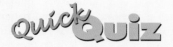

Quick Quiz

1) What is the cause *and* treatment of a high-volume hyponatremic patient? Low volume?

2) Which drugs can cause SIADH?

3) How do you treat SIADH?

4) How do you differentiate between SIADH and psychogenic polydipsia?

5) What can induce central pontine myelinolysis?

6) How do you treat severe hypernatremia?

7) How does measured ADH change in central vs. nephrogenic DI?

HYPERNATREMIA

Overview

Severe hypernatremia is fairly rare, but always represents a water deficit. It doesn't occur unless the patient is unable to get to water (debilitated or H_2O unavailable) or the thirst mechanism is defective. Unlike hyponatremia, these patients are always hyperosmolar, so the first step is determining volume status. Low volume implies high water loss and some Na^+ loss (of course, more water than Na^+ is lost).

Treat severe hypernatremia with normal saline first to correct the hypotension and/or volume depletion, and only then with hypotonic fluids to further correct the hypernatremia. Remember, even isotonic saline is lower in tonicity than hyperosmolar serum, and it would be correcting the tonicity and depleted volume. Normal saline is especially necessary in patients with hyperosmolar hyperglycemia.

The amount of free water needed in a hypernatremic patient is calculated by multiplying the total body water (60% of weight in kg) by the fractional difference between patient's Na^+ and normal Na^+.

$$Vol_{water} = (total\ body\ water)\ (Na^+_{serum} - 145)/145$$
$$Vol_{water} = .6(body\ weight)\ (Na^+_{serum} - 145)/145$$

So, if a 100 kg patient has a serum Na^+ of 156, the amount of free water needed is 4.5 liters. This is usually given over 1–2 days. This is meant to decrease the sodium concentration at a rate of 0.5 mEq/L/hr. See pg 4-14 for causes of volume contraction.

High volume—this is unusual and typically not serious. It most often occurs with mineralocorticoid excess (1° hyperaldosteronism). Usually, the only time a serious result occurs is after giving large amounts of sodium bicarbonate during ACLS. Treat with loop diuretics and free water.

Normal volume—from decreased free water intake with diabetes insipidus (DI). Think of central DI in the patient with high Na^+ and high urine volume who also has a history of recent neurosurgery, head trauma, or brain cancer/brain metastases. Otherwise, it is usually nephrogenic.

Water Restriction Test

The water restriction test not only diagnoses DI, but also differentiates between the 2 types of DI. In a healthy person, when plasma osmolality increases to 295, ADH level is high and urine osmolality is maximally concentrated (> 700 mOsm/L). More on this in the Endocrinology section.

• In central DI, even with water restriction, the ADH stays low and the urine unconcentrated. Giving extra ADH (vasopressin or desmopressin [DDAVP]) quickly increases the urine concentration. Use chlorpropamide to treat partial central DI.

• In nephrogenic DI, the ADH is appropriately high, but the urine is not concentrated. Giving extra ADH does not increase the concentration of the urine. Treat nephrogenic DI with thiazide diuretics.

Remember: High ADH (from SIADH) causes hyponatremia with normal volume. Low ADH (from DI) causes hypernatremia, also with normal volume!

Urine Osmolality

Urinary osmolality can range from 40–1400 mOsm/L. To make sense of the osmolality, you must also know the urine output (liters/d). Multiply the osmolality x output (1 kg = 1 liter) to get total osmoles output per day. Normal is about 500. This is important in the case of a patient with high Na^+ and high urine output. If the 24-hour solute output is > 900 mOsm, think of an osmotic cause of the hypernatremia (e.g., hyperglycemia); whereas in DI, the 24-hour osmoles is normal, so the urine is very dilute.

DIURETICS, RTA, AND NORMAL RENAL PHYSIOLOGY

PROXIMAL TUBULE

We will now discuss aspects of normal renal function and the effects on the tubules by diuretics. Refer to Figure 4-1 and Figure 4-2 during this discussion. Consider the entire text in this discussion to be highlighted—i.e., "must know"!

Proximal convoluted tubule (PCT): 90% of the HCO_3^- (bicarbonate) is resorbed here by means of several chemical changes. The resorption process is driven by H^+ being secreted! This makes homeostatic sense: Acidosis causes increased H^+ secretion and, therefore, increased HCO_3^- resorption. H^+ combines with HCO_3^- to form H_2CO_3 (carbonic acid) which, with the help of carbonic anhydrase in the brush border of the proximal tubule, is converted to $H_2O + CO_2$. The CO_2 is absorbed into the cells and again, with the help of carbonic anhydrase, is converted to HCO_3^-. Although this is represented in the diagram, it is better explained here in the text. A carbonic anhydrase inhibitor (acetazolamide [Diamox®]) causes diuresis with bicarbonate wasting, resulting in a metabolic acidosis just like proximal (Type II) RTA.

Calcium is also absorbed in the proximal tubule. When treating severe hypercalcemia, normal saline is infused at a high rate along with a loop diuretic. The saline expands the volume

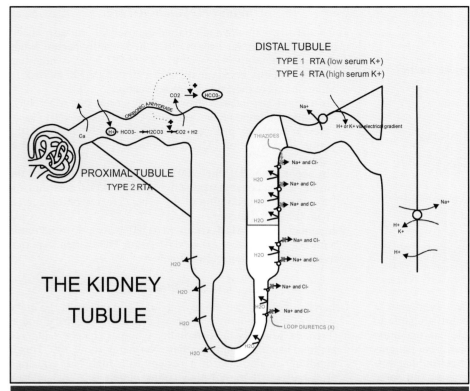

DISTAL TUBULE

TYPE 1 RTA (low serum K+)
TYPE 4 RTA (high serum K+)

PROXIMAL TUBULE
TYPE 2 RTA

THE KIDNEY
TUBULE

Figure 4-1: The Renal Tubule – Basic Physiology

Both furosemide and bumetanide contain sulfa, so use ethacrynic acid if the patient has a sulfa allergy.

DISTAL TUBULE

The distal tubule is where Na^+ is actively resorbed, and H^+ in the form of salts (NH_4^+ or phosphate salts) and K^+ are then excreted—flowing back down the electrical gradient created by the active resorption of Na^+. This effect used to be called the Na^+-K^+ pump, but actually it is the "Na^+ pump and K^+/H^+ electrical excretion gradient" (you might think up a better name than this!). Functionally, there is a "molar" competition between the secretion of H^+ and K^+. When there is a metabolic acidosis, more H^+ is excreted in preference to K^+ (acidosis also causes a shift of K^+ out of the body's cells), causing a tendency toward hyperkalemia. Conversely, hyperkalemia can cause an acidosis by the same means. Aldosterone facilitates this active resorption of Na^+ and, therefore, the excretion of K^+ and H^+. In the person not on drugs, virtually all the K^+ appearing in the urine is due to distal secretion.

and causes an increased flow in the proximal tubule that prevents calcium resorption, and the greatly increased calcium load then delivered to the distal tubule overwhelms the distal tubule's ability to absorb calcium, while its ability to absorb is blocked by the loop diuretic, so a calciuresis ensues.

LOOP OF HENLE:

As the tubular fluid progresses down the (descending) loop of Henle, free H_2O is "sucked out" of the fluid following the osmotic gradient (the renal medulla is very hypertonic—[why?]). At the base of the loop, the tubular fluid is maximally concentrated. In the ascending limb, 25% of the filtered NaCl is actively absorbed, and the permeability is decreased so H_2O is unable to follow—diluting the tubular fluid. This active pumping out of the NaCl also increases the hypertonicity of the medulla [that's why!] and causes H_2O from the descending limb to effectively "follow" the Na^+ out of the ascending limb (think about this a minute, and be sure you "get it" before you move on).

Blockage of this absorption of Na^+ in the ascending loop with loop diuretics results in diuresis. The loop diuretics are furosemide (Lasix®), bumetanide (Bumex®), torsemide (Demadex®), and ethacrynic acid (Edecrin®). Loop diuretics remain effective even when GFR is low—i.e., CrCl < 20. Loop diuretics also increase Ca^+ excretion.

COLLECTING DUCT

The collecting duct is where ADH has its effect. In the normal kidney, the urine is very dilute by the time it reaches the collecting duct. ADH increases the permeability of the collecting duct to water, allowing the free water to resorb into the hypertonic renal medulla. When there is no ADH, a very dilute urine is produced.

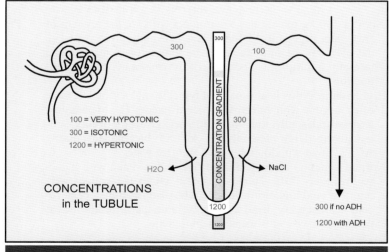

Figure 4-2: Osmolar Concentrations in the Renal Tubule

notes

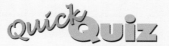

DIURETICS – NOTES TO KNOW!

Spironolactone is an aldosterone antagonist, so it is K^+-sparing and hence, also can cause acidosis.

On the other hand, diuretics that act in the early distal tubule increase the Na^+ load to the distal tubule, where resultant increased Na^+ uptake results in increased K^+ excretion (…this is it! Remember this, and you will always remember why you lose K^+ with loop diuretics and thiazides).

Triamterene and amiloride are K^+-sparing because they inhibit Na^+ entry into the distal cells and thereby block the K^+ and H^+ secretory process.

Thiazides decrease the Na^+ and Cl^- absorption at the early distal convoluted tubule and cortical thick ascending limb, after much of the filtered NaCl has been reabsorbed in the PCT and ascending limb. Thiazides are not effective at a low GFR—i.e., CrCl < 20. Thiazides have a longer half-life than loop diuretics and, unlike loop diuretics, thiazides decrease Ca^+ excretion.

Combined with a strong loop diuretic, thiazides in low doses have a synergistic effect on excretion. So when furosemide is maxed out, adding a low dose of a thiazide is often effective!

RENAL TUBULAR ACIDOSIS

RTA is a normal anion gap (i.e., hyperchloremic—see pg 4-2) metabolic acidosis, usually caused by a defect—often genetic—in renal tubule function. There is one proximal type (Type 2) and two distal types (Types 1 and 4). Type 3 previously described a distal RTA that is now considered a subset of Type 1. Now the term Type 3 generally refers to a very rare autosomal recessive (AR) lack of carbonic anhydrase II (it won't be discussed here).

Serum K^+ level is low-to-normal in Types 1 and 2, and high in Type 4. Note: On the boards, expect to have Type 1 and 2 RTA patients presenting with a low serum K^+.

Type 1 RTA (Distal RTA) is a distal defect in which there is a problem with H^+ secretion. Serum H^+ builds up, and the patients become acidotic. K^+, instead of H^+, follows the anions out instead of H^+, and hypokalemia sometimes is the result.

Type 1 RTA is commonly associated with hypercalciuria. The major causes are:
- autoimmune disorders (Sjögren, SLE, and rheumatoid arthritis)
- hereditary hypercalciuria, hyperparathyroidism, and Vit D intoxication.

Other causes include:
- drugs (amphotericin B, lithium)
- hypergammaglobulinemia (e.g., chronic hepatitis)

Type 1 RTA commonly causes renal stones—probably from a decreased citrate excretion and hypercalciuria.

Treatment is usually alkali therapy and addressing the cause.

Type 2 RTA (Proximal RTA) is caused by a mechanism similar to that of acetazolamide—bicarbonate wasting in the proximal tubule. [Know:] Even though there is bicarbonate wasting in Type 2 RTA, once the serum bicarbonate is low enough (i.e., the serum is acidic enough), H^+ once again starts secreting in the proximal tubule, causing the resorption of bicarbonate. Early in Type 2, the urine pH is very high, but the acid-base metabolism quickly re-equilibrates to the lower bicarb threshold, and an acidic urine (i.e., normal values) is usually found with diagnosis of Type 2 RTA.

Type 2 RTA is usually caused by:
- multiple myeloma
- carbonic anhydrase drugs, like acetazolamide

Other causes are:
- other drugs (amphotericin B and 6-mercaptopurine)
- heavy metal poisonings (lead, copper, mercury, cadmium)
- amyloidosis
- disorders of protein/carbohydrate/amino acid metabolism

Note: Fanconi syndrome is generalized proximal tubule dysfunction, which can be caused by just about any disorder or drug that causes Type 2 RTA—especially MM and acetazolamide. Fanconi syndrome patients additionally have proximal loss of phosphorus, uric acid, glucose, and amino acids that shows up as hypophosphatemia, hypouricosuria, and renal glycosuria (glucosuria with normal serum glucose level). So look for Type 2 RTA in patients with these other findings.

Idiopathic Type 2 RTA can often be treated with Na^+ restriction alone.

Type 4 RTA can be the result of aldosterone deficiency or due to distal tubule resistance to aldosterone, impairing the function of the Na^+/K^+-H^+ (cation) exchange mechanism. The Na^+ no longer exchanges normally with H^+ or K^+, causing acidemia and hyperkalemia.

Table 4-5: Renal Tubular Acidoses (RTAs)

A COMPARISON of the RTAs Note: All have normal anion gap (hyperchloremic) metabolic acidosis						
	Metabolic Acidosis	Urine pH	Serum K$^+$	Renal Stones	Mechanism	Main Causes
Type 1 Distal RTA	Yes	> 5.5*	low-nl	Yes*	Decreased H$^+$ secretion in DISTAL tubule (H$^+$ builds up in blood, K$^+$ secreted instead of H$^+$ causing low serum H)	Autoimmune (SLE, Sjögren) Hereditary hypercalciuria, hyperparathyroidism, Vit D overdose Drugs (amphotericin B, Lithium) Hypergammaglobulinemia
Type 2 Proximal RTA	Yes	< 5.5, although high initially	low-nl	No	Decreased resorption of HCO$_3^-$ from PROXIMAL tubule (bicarbonate wasting leaves net H$^+$ excess)	MM, Acetazolamide use, Cystinosis, Heavy metal poisonings Amyloidosis, Disorders of protein/carbohydrate/amino acid metabolism Remember Fanconi syndrome**!
Type 4	Yes	< 5.5	HIGH ****	No	Decreased cation exchange in DISTAL tubule (decr'd H$^+$ and K$^+$ secretion cause plasma buildup of H$^+$ and K$^+$)	Diabetic nephropathy, Spironolactone Aldosterone deficiency, Obstructive uropathy, Interstitial nephritis, Renal transplant

Clues for Diagnosis:
    * Type 1: High urine pH consistently occurs in type 1 RTA. Also suspect type 1 with renal stones or hypercalciuria.
    ** Type 2: Suspect type 2 RTA if patient presents with Fanconi syndrome. Urine pH is high only initially.
    **** Type 4: High K$^+$ occurs only in type 4 RTA.

Type 4 RTA is usually a result of:
- diabetic nephropathy (main cause), causing hyporeninemic hypoaldosteronism.
- spironolactone
- interstitial nephritis
- obstructive uropathy
- renal transplant

Although it makes theoretical sense to treat this cause of Type 4 RTA with fludrocortisone (Florinef®; a synthetic adrenocortical steroid with very potent mineralocorticoid effect), this often leads to too much fluid retention.

Dietary restriction of sodium may be sufficient treatment. Otherwise, give furosemide—a commonly used, effective treatment. Note that NSAIDs can decrease the renin output even more and exacerbate the hyperkalemia.

Review: Clues to type of RTA [Know!]:
All have a normal anion gap metabolic acidosis.
Type 1: Associated with renal stones and hypercalciuria. High urine pH despite a metabolic acidosis.
Type 2: Think acetazolamide and bicarbonate wasting. If a patient presents with Fanconi syndrome, remember to check if they have Type 2 RTA.

Type 4: Think aldosterone deficiency and hyperkalemia.

The Board exam questions and answers concerning RTA may not even mention RTA. Often, the patient presents with a history of nephrocalcinosis/diabetes/heavy metal poisoning /MM, etc., and you are supposed to pick out the most likely serum and urine chemistry, or the best treatment based on serum and urine chemistry.

After reviewing Table 4-5, do the following questions that refer to Table 4-6.

Table 4-6: RTAs—Serum and Urine Chemistry

	PLASMA				URINE		
	Na$^+$	K$^+$	Cl$^-$	CO$_2$	pH	K$^+$	Na$^+$
Normal	135-145	3.5-5	95-105	22-30	variable	25-100	100-260
A	140	2.6	113	17	7.9	50	100
B	140	5.5	117	13	6	50	100
C	140	4.0	115	15	6	50	100
D	140	4.0	105	15	6	50	100
E	140	4.0	115	15	6	10	10
F	130	4.0	117	13	6	50	100

notes

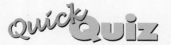

Quick Quiz

1) Diabetic nephropathy causes which type RTA?
2) What is often the simplest treatment for type 4 RTA?
3) Know Table 4-5 and Table 4-6!
4) Addison disease causes what type of potassium abnormality?
5) What is the immediate treatment for severe hyperkalemia?

What chemistry profile, A thru F, in Table 4-6 fits the following?
1) DKA patient
2) diabetic patient with renal insufficiency
3) patient with MM
4) woman with renal stones
5) patient with heavy metal poisoning
6) patient with severe diarrhea

Here is one approach to analyzing a table like this:
✓ First, peruse the values and, noticing that all of the CO_2 (more correctly HCO_3^-) values are low, say "Oh yeah, this must be one of those RTA problems."
✓ Next, look for any with a high anion gap (usually normal Cl) or a very low urine sodium, since these are red herrings and not RTAs. Label these, and we will get to them at the end.
✓ Next, look for a urine that is not acidic (> 6.0) despite the low CO_2. Ensure that there is also a low-to-normal serum K^+ and label it "high urine pH—Type 1—autoimmune, calcium."
✓ Next, look for a high K^+, and label it "Type 4—diabetic nephropathy, spironolactone."
✓ Then, label the (probably) last one "Type 2— MM, Fanconi, heavy metal, amino acids."
Note: All of the above have a low CO_2 and high Cl^- (i.e., normal anion gap).
The metabolic acidosis with low urine sodium is almost certainly diarrhea-induced volume contraction. The high anion gap acidosis could be ethylene glycol, methanol, lactic/ketoacidosis, or salicylates. And what if you see a low anion gap? This means there is probably some artifactual lowering of the Na^+. This occurs in hyperlipidemia and multiple myeloma. I suspect that it would be in a MM patient with Type 2 RTA chemistry.
Correct answers are 1) D; 2) B; 3) C; 4) A; 5) C; 6) E.

MINERALS
POTASSIUM

Overview

Potassium: Normally, even slight hyperkalemia stimulates the release of aldosterone which, if the kidneys are functioning normally, causes increased absorption of Na^+ distally and, therefore, increased excretion of K^+ (and H^+) in the distal collecting duct.

Alkalosis, insulin, beta-agonists, and aldosterone stimulate an increased uptake of K^+ by cells (thereby decreasing serum K^+). Acidosis and alpha-agonists inhibit uptake.

All excretion of K^+ takes place in the distal tubule (remember that all of the filtered K^+ is resorbed in the proximal tubule). Decreased urinary Na^+ and decreased urine output from renal failure also cause an increase in K^+ retention.

Hyperkalemia

Hyperkalemia is caused by
• decreased excretion (drugs, renal failure, hypoaldosteronism—e.g., Addison disease),
• increased production (trauma, tumor lysis), and
• hypertonic states, such as hyperglycemia (the K^+ follows the free water out of the cells).

Drugs are probably the most common cause of hyperkalemia; main culprits are ACEI/ARBs and beta-blockers—especially if the patient has normal or increased intake of K^+.

In the patient with high K^+ from hyporeninemic hypoaldosteronism (kidney problem), avoid NSAIDs, ACEI/ARBs, beta-blockers, and heparin. Note that you should not empirically give comatose diabetics D_{50} without first checking blood glucose with a fingerstick glucometer. If these patients are in DKA, they may already have a high K^+ (from hyperglycemia and acidosis); giving IV glucose only exacerbates the hyperkalemia. High K^+ itself can cause or exacerbate metabolic acidosis by competing with the renal H^+ excretion.

Treatment of hyperkalemia: The cardiac effects of hyperkalemia are due to the large difference between intracellular and extracellular K^+ levels. Initiate treatment in hyperkalemic patients if the K^+ > 7.0, or if there are ECG changes (high peaked T waves; then prolonged PR; then loss of the P wave). Treatment: IV calcium, insulin and glucose, $NaHCO_3$, and K^+ binding resins.

Immediate treatment: IV calcium: either 1 amp calcium chloride or 3 amps of calcium gluconate. Within 5 minutes, IV calcium counters the effect of the high K^+ on the heart. Then give insulin and glucose, which increases entry of K^+ into cells—onset is 15–30 minutes, duration 12–24 hours. Then give $NaHCO_3$ (shifts K^+ into the cells—onset is within 15–45 minutes, duration 12–24 hours), and K^+ binding resins.

K^+ binding resin, given as a retention enema, starts working in 30 minutes and actually removes K^+, while the others push K^+ into the cells—with a shift back out the moment you turn your back!

notes

Remember: The hyperkalemic ECG changes are peaked T waves, widened QRS, and severe bradyarrhythmias.

Hypokalemia

With persistent K^+ loss from body stores, serum K^+ level does not decrease to below normal until there is a net loss of 200–300 mEq. Therefore, large amounts of KCl are usually required for treatment. Remember, severe hypokalemia may cause U waves, decreased deep tendon reflexes, and rhabdomyolysis.

Causes of hypokalemia:
   1) diuretics (most common)
   2) hyperaldosteronism
   3) high insulin
   4) GI loss
   5) Type 1 RTA
   6) drugs (e.g., gentamicin→renal wasting of K+)
   7) genetic: Bartter syndrome, Gitelman syndrome, and Liddle syndrome.

Let's discuss these a little:

Hypokalemia is usually caused by diuretics. There is telltale high K^+ and Cl^- in the urine.

If the hypokalemic patient is hypertensive and has no history of diuretic use, consider hyperaldosteronism. ~ 40% of patients with hypertension and hypokalemia of no obvious cause have hyperaldosteronism!! Hyperaldosteronism is either primary or secondary (from renovascular HTN). Primary hyperaldosteronism leads to hyporeninemia and a high BP and low K^+. Renovascular HTN causes a hyperreninemic hyperaldosteronism (decreased renal blood flow from renal artery stenosis → increased renin → increased angiotensin II → increased aldosterone).

How do you differentiate 1° from 2° hyperaldosteronism? Give 2 liters of normal saline IV over 3–4 hours—non-suppression of the aldosterone level indicates primary hyperaldosteronism. On the other hand, suppression indicates secondary hyperaldosteronism (usually due to renovascular hypertension), and you must do a renal arteriogram [see pg 4-17]).

K^+ redistribution into the cells results from alkalosis, insulin, or glucose administration (and 2° endogenous insulin production).

Type 1 distal RTA is another possible cause. In Type 1 RTA, there is a hypokalemic, hyperchloremic acidosis with renal wasting of K^+ (RTA—see pg 4-9).

Hypokalemia can also be caused by gastrointestinal K^+ loss from diarrhea, laxative abuse, and fistulas.

Vomiting can cause both alkalosis and hyperreninemic hyperaldosteronism.

Gentamicin can cause renal K^+ wasting, along with magnesium wasting. Hypomagnesemia is often an associated finding in patients with hypokalemia; it is caused by the same mechanism that causes the low K^+.

Bartter syndrome is usually an autosomal recessive disorder in which there is abnormal NaCl transport in the thick ascending limb of the loop of Henle, leading to K^+, Na^+, and Cl^- wasting. Gitelman syndrome is like a milder form of Bartter's, but with the additional component of low-urine calcium (this is used to distinguish it from Bartter syndrome). Both cause hypokalemic metabolic alkalosis. Liddle syndrome is a rare cause of hypertension and hypokalemia in which there is primary Na^+ retention, so both renin and aldosterone levels are low.

Treat hypokalemia by removing the known cause (if any and if able to) and giving oral potassium supplements. Poor response usually means the deficit is large, and the patient merely requires more potassium.

CALCIUM

Regulation of calcium: PTH and vitamin D metabolites cause changes in the way kidney, GI, and bone handle calcium (more in the Endocrinology section). Calcium circulates in an inactive, bound form (usually with albumin) and an active, ionized/unbound form. With hypoalbuminemia, only the bound form decreases; the ionized calcium level does not decrease. For each decrease in albumin of 1, the total calcium decreases by .7, yet the ionized calcium level remains the same, so there is no effect on the body. In pregnancy, there is increased calcium absorption and excretion, because the active form of vitamin D, 1,25-$(OH)_2$-D3, is > 2 x normal.

Hypercalcemia found incidentally in an asymptomatic patient is usually due to 1° hyperparathyroidism (especially consider if there is a history of neck irradiation). On the other hand, hypercalcemia found in inpatients or in patients undergoing a cancer workup is usually due to cancer.

Furosemide increases calcium excretion and is used to treat hypercalcemia. For severe hypercalcemia, give 1–2 liters of normal saline at ~ 300 cc/hr, along with the furosemide. This causes a rapid decrease of serum calcium.

Hypocalcemia may be caused by hypoparathyroidism, pseudohypoparathyroidism, hypomagnesemia, rhabdomyolysis, acute or chronic renal failure, and severe pancreatitis. Renal failure results in a decreased renal conversion of 1-OH-D3 to the active 1,25-$(OH)_2$-D3 (so there is an increased PTH in these patients).

Thiazide diuretics indirectly decrease calcium excretion in the urine. They are used to treat hypocalcemia caused by hypercalciuria. More on this in the Endocrinology section.

Treatment: Hypercalcemia: saline and furosemide. Hypocalcemia: calcium with vitamin D.

MAGNESIUM

Hypermagnesemia is rare and occurs from the use of:
   • Mg-containing laxatives or antacids in patients with renal failure, and
   • MgSO4 over-infusion during eclampsia.

Do not give magnesium-citrate bowel prep in a patient with renal failure.

Symptoms begin when magnesium level is > 4–6 mEq/L: There is initially nausea, followed by sedation, muscle weakness,

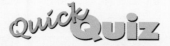

and a loss of deep tendon reflexes, progressing to paralysis (including heart and respiratory muscles).

Treatment: Treat acute symptoms with volume expansion to induce a diuresis and calcium to treat symptoms. Hemodialysis is necessary in renal failure.

Hypomagnesemia is, on the other hand, very common. Causes:
- amphotericin B
- cisplatin
- insulin
- alcohol withdrawal
- loop diuretics
- pentamidine
- hungry bone syndrome
- gentamicin
- cyclosporine

Hypomagnesemia can be caused by renal wasting or redistribution. Renal wasting is usually caused by diuretics (especially loop). Gentamicin and cisplatin can cause a renal wasting of magnesium, which, in both cases, persists after the drug is stopped. Redistribution occurs in alcohol withdrawal, insulin administration, and in hungry bone syndrome (after parathyroidectomy, the bones "suck up" Ca and Mg). Pentamidine and cyclosporine also commonly cause hypomagnesemia.

Low magnesium level itself causes decreased calcium and K^+, so always check for a low magnesium in patients presenting with hypocalcemia and/or hypokalemia, because these deficiencies are not correctable until magnesium stores (not just the serum level!) are replenished!

Refractory cardiac arrhythmias are associated with depleted magnesium stores (even with normal serum levels!). Magnesium is receiving intense scrutiny now. The standard recommendation for parenteral Mg is 12 ml of 50% $MgSO_4$ (49 mEq) in 1 L D_5W over 3 hours, followed by 80 mEq in 2 L D_5W over the next 21 hours. For less severe cases, use oral Mg oxide.

PHOSPHATE

Hyperphosphatemia—acute increase can be from:
- acute tubular necrosis—especially with rhabdomyolysis
- IV solutions
- tumor lysis after chemotherapy

Chronic increase of phosphate is seen in:
- hypoparathyroidism
- chronic kidney disease

If the PO_4 is > 5.5 mg/dL, treat with calcium-containing antacids, which bind PO_4 in the gut if the calcium is low, with sevelamer (Renagel®), or lanthanum (Fosrenol®) if the Ca x Phos product is > 55. Sevelamer and lanthanum decrease phosphate levels without the concern for calcium accumulation.

Hypophosphatemia—Think "alcoholism" and alcoholic ketoacidosis! If severe (PO_4 is < 1 mg/dL), it may cause rhabdomyolysis (as can low K^+), cardiomyopathy, respiratory insufficiency with failure of diaphragm function, and nervous system problems initially consisting of irritability and hyperventilation, then profound muscle weakness, then seizures, coma, and death.

Chronic malnutrition (as in alcoholics) results in increased catabolic release of phosphate, which then gets excreted by the kidneys, depleting total body stores. Even though these patients may have a normal phosphate level on admission, they may become symptomatic (extreme muscle weakness) a few days after a normal diet is established because, as the glycogen level is returned to normal, the muscle cells become anabolic and take up phosphate, thereby reducing serum levels. Alcoholic patients with hepatic encephalopathy often have a respiratory alkalosis and may receive glucose solutions, both of which cause phosphate to enter cells, in turn causing severe hypophosphatemia, which may precipitate acute rhabdomyolysis.

Other causes of severe hypophosphatemia include phosphate-binding antacids, DKA, and "re-feeding" malnourished patients (hyperal in the ICU). Refeeding syndrome occurs when severely malnourished patients are fed high carbohydrate loads. Refeeding is discussed in Pulmonary Medicine → Critical Care → Nutritional Support.

Table 4-7: Volume Contraction—Serum and Urine Chemistry					
Volume Contraction	**Serum Na^+**	**Serum Cl^-**	**Serum Bicarb**	**Urine Cl^-**	**Calculated Urine Osmo**
Vomiting	nl	95	35	10	700
Diarrhea	nl	115	15	10	700
Thiazides	-	95	35	100	700
Osmotic Diuresis	-	nl	nl	100	300 (but high volume)

notes

Treatment: Give supplemental phosphate to patients with DKA or those having alcohol withdrawal; it should be included in hyperalimentation fluid.

Patients with reduced renal function require less supplemental phosphate; phosphate supplementation may actually cause severe hyperphosphatemia!

VOLUME CONTRACTION

Look for the following, unique combination of factors in the answers to exam questions asking about volume contraction states. See Table 4-7.

Vomiting (especially frequent, surreptitious vomiting) causes: metabolic alkalosis
- low serum Cl^- (losing stomach HCl in the emesis—makes sense)
- hypokalemia from renal K^+ wasting

Diarrhea causes metabolic acidosis and an appropriately high serum Cl^- (HCl increases as bicarbonate is lost in the stool).

Thiazide diuretics, like vomiting, cause a metabolic alkalosis with low serum Cl^- but, unlike vomiting, cause a high Cl^- in the urine—(effectively losing HCl in the urine). The actual mechanism is: Thiazides cause more NaCl to be delivered distally, where more Na^+ is then available for reabsorption and, therefore, there is increased H^+ and K^+ excretion (see the discussion on pg 4-9). So there actually is increased HCl, NaCl, and KCl in the urine. Okay! Review the logic here, and you will always remember these points!

All of the above have concentrated urine. On the other hand, osmotic diuresis (mannitol, hyperglycemia) causes a high urine output with a normal urine osmolality, and thus increased solute loss per day.

Remember: Diabetes insipidus (nephrogenic or neurogenic) tends to cause hypernatremia and volume contraction, but the patient can have a normal intravascular volume and sodium if water intake is sufficient—so it is only the patients who are unable to drink who become hypernatremic.

Lithium impairs the kidney's concentrating ability and effectively produces a nephrogenic diabetes insipidus.

EDEMA

When a patient has primary hyperaldosteronism (i.e., hyporeninemic), there is no peripheral edema (barring other factors). Patients with secondary hyperaldosteronism due to cirrhosis, CHF, or nephrotic syndrome often develop edema. Why is that? Answer: 2/3 of the filtered sodium and water is passively resorbed in the proximal tubule. With primary hyperaldosteronism, and because of the increased sodium and therefore total body water, less is absorbed in the proximal tubule—somewhat counterbalancing the effects of aldosterone on the distal tubule. Patients with CHF, cirrhosis, and low albumin, have a decreased effective intravascular volume (as seen by the kidney). This stimulates both the renin-angiotensin system and increases the amount of proximal

tubular absorption. The resultant increase in total body water causes edema.

HYPERTENSION

NOTE

Much of the following is adapted from the JNC 7 (7th report from the Joint National Committee on Prevention, Evaluation, and Treatment of Hypertension) published in 2003. This can be downloaded from the web:
http://www.nhlbi.nih.gov/guidelines/hypertension/

PRIMARY HTN

95% of all HTN is primary (i.e., essential, idiopathic). The systolic blood pressure (SBP) and diastolic blood pressure (DBP) define the stages of HTN:

Stage I: SBP 140–159 or DBP 90–99
Stage II: SBP $\geq$ 160 or DBP $\geq$ 100—Averaged from $\geq$ 2 readings taken from each of $\geq$ 2 visits after the initial screening.

In any of these stages, morbidity and mortality are higher for men than women, and higher for blacks than whites. HTN itself is also more frequent in blacks than whites. This may be due to a decreased Na^+ excretion. HTN is well correlated with obesity in young persons.

Of course, primary hypertension does have causes—they just have not yet been discovered.

Hyperinsulinemia has been getting much attention and coverage the last several years. It was found that obese patients with decreased glucose tolerance and HTN have an insulin resistance that causes hyperinsulinemia, which (theoretically, at least) causes, or is associated with, volume retention, vascular hypertrophy, and sympathetic overactivity which, in turn, cause HTN ("Syndrome X").

Table 4-8: Identifiable Causes of Hypertension	
IF YOU FIND THIS:	THINK THIS:
Truncal obesity with purple striae	Cushing syndrome
Labile HTN	Pheochromocytoma
Abdominal bruits, esp if in renal area or have diastolic component (i.e. continuous)	Renovascular HTN
Decreased BP in lower extremities or absent/delayed femoral pulses	Coarctation of the aorta
Abdominal or flank masses	Polycystic kidneys
Elevated creatinine or abnormal urinalysis	Renal parenchymal disease
Hypercalcemia	Hyperparathyroidism
Hypokalemia	Primary hyperaldosteronism

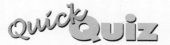

1) Which patients should you be very careful about giving supplemental phosphates to, even if they have low-serum levels?

2) State the cutoffs for the different stages of HTN.

3) A newly diagnosed patient with HTN presents and has a systolic epigastric bruit. Does this finding by itself warrant further workup?

4) What is the most common cause of secondary HTN?

5) Thiazides are effective antihypertensive agents only if they are coupled with what?

If the diastolic blood pressure is < 85, recheck it in 2–3 years. If 85–90, recheck it in 1 year. If 90–104, recheck within 2 months. If 105–114, work up within 2 weeks. If > 115, work up immediately.

EVALUATION OF HTN

This is the standard evaluation for newly diagnosed hypertension (as above). Initially, you look for reversible causes of hypertension. See Table 4-8.

History: Ask about history or symptoms of CAD, PVD, cerebrovascular disease, renal disease, DM, and lipid problems. Family history or symptoms of the same. Use of alcohol, smoking, street drugs, prescribed meds; diet history; psychosocial history.

Full physical exam including:

General: height, weight, and waist size. Extremities: 2 BP checks (with verification in the other arm), other extremities for decreased pulses, bruits, and edema. Head: funduscopic for hypertensive changes. Neck: bruits, enlarged thyroid. Chest: rales, wheezes. Full heart auscultation. Abd: abnormal masses, bruits, abnormal pulsations.

Initial lab tests for all hypertensive patients: serum chemistry (K^+, Na^+, Ca^{+2}, creatinine, fasting glucose, total cholesterol, HDL cholesterol), U/A, and a 12-lead ECG.

Indications for further evaluation for secondary causes of HTN include abnormal initial lab tests, an abrupt onset, age < 30 years, malignant HTN, refractory HTN, hypercalcemia, hypokalemia with kaliuresis, systolic-diastolic bruits in the epigastrium or lateralizing over a kidney (systolic bruits alone are not an indication). Secondary HTN comprises only 5% of HTN cases.

Renovascular HTN causing a secondary hyperaldosteronism is the most common cause of secondary HTN. Other less-common-to-rare causes are Cushing syndrome, coarctation of the aorta, primary aldosteronism, thyroid/parathyroid dis-

ease, chronic kidney disease, sleep apnea, drug-induced, and pheochromocytoma.

DRUGS FOR HTN

Diuretics—As mentioned before (pg 4-9), thiazides are not effective if CrCl is < 20. Loop diuretics do work at a CrCl < 20, and they have a short duration of action, so give twice per day. To decrease hypokalemia, encourage the patient on diuretics to use moderate dietary salt, because both high and low sodium ingestion increases the tendency for hypokalemia! Give K^+ supplementation with the diuretics if $K^+ < 3.5$, the patient is on digoxin, has glucose intolerance, or has cardiac disease. Diuretics, especially thiazide, are effective only if coupled with dietary Na^+ restriction.

Beta-blockers decrease cardiac output, sympathetic tone, and renin production. Each one differs by 3 factors: amount of lipid solubility, cardioselectivity, and sympathomimetic activity. See Table 4-9.

Metoprolol (Lopressor®) and propranolol (Inderal®) are lipid-soluble. Increased lipid solubility means shorter half-life (with increased first-pass effect) and easier passage through the blood-brain barrier. Atenolol (Tenormin®) and nadolol (Corgard®) are the least lipid-soluble, and so have fewer CNS side effects and longer half-lives. The agonist effect of pindolol (Visken®) is in contrast to the bradycardic effect caused by the others shown here. The beta-1 selectivity of metoprolol and atenolol is lost at high doses!

Consider avoiding beta-blockers in patients with reactive airway disease, hyperlipidemia, and PVD; and avoid diuretics in patients with gout, hyperlipidemia, and orthostatic hypotension.

Brief review: renin-angiotensin-aldosterone system. Renin is a protease released from the kidney in response to decreased blood pressure and decreased extracellular fluid volume (ECF). Renin converts angiotensinogen to angiotensin I. Angiotensin I is converted to angiotensin II by means of proteolytic enzymes, including angiotensin-converting enzyme

Table 4-9: Characteristics of Beta-Blocker Antihypertensive Drugs				
BETA-BLOCKERS		Lipid solubility	Cardio (beta-1) selectivity	Beta-1 agonist activity
Atenolol	(Tenormin)	-	+++	-
Metoprolol	(Lopressor)	++	+++	-
Nadolol	(Corgard)	-	-	-
Pindolol	(Visken)	+	-	+
Propranolol	(Inderal)	+++	-	-
Timolol	(Blocadren)	+	-	-

Note: All names in parentheses are registered brand names

notes

(ACE). Angiotensin II increases blood pressure by direct vasoconstriction, potentiation of the sympathetic nervous system, and stimulation of aldosterone synthesis with consequent sodium and water retention.

ACE inhibitors (ACEI: captopril, enalapril, benazepril, fosinopril, lisinopril, quinapril, ramipril, imidapril, perindopril, trandolapril) inhibit conversion of angiotensin I to II, causing a decrease in angiotensin II and, hence, in aldosterone, while angiotensin receptor blockers (ARBs) act similarly at the angiotensin II receptor level. In the kidney, both result in a decreased tone of the efferent loop of the glomerulus, which causes a decrease in glomerular capillary pressure. This decreased glomerular pressure results in a decrease of the progression of both diabetic and hypertensive nephropathies, and other types of chronic kidney disease.

Angiotensin II receptor blockers (ARBs: losartan, irbesartan, candesartan, valsartan, olmesartan) exert effects similar to ACE inhibitors, and are recommended for use in diabetics and patients with indications for ACE inhibitors but who are unable to tolerate them, usually due to cough.

ACEI and ARBs are the drugs of choice for mild-to-moderate HTN in patients with diabetic nephropathy. There are minimal CNS or sexual function side effects. They are most effective if renin is high or normal.

When not to give ACEI/ARBs: Do not give to pregnant patients (teratogenic). Because hyperkalemia is usually due to decreased renal K^+ excretion, avoid ACEI/ARBs in hyperkalemic patients; they may worsen the hyperkalemia. You must use ACE inhibitors with caution in patients with bilateral renal-artery obstruction (> 70%) or severe CHF because, by decreasing the GFR, the prerenal azotemia found in these conditions worsens. ACE inhibitors are contraindicated in any low-renin diseases.

Calcium-channel blockers—more on these in the Cardiology section. They are most effective if the renin is low (ACE inhibitors best if renin is high or normal)!

TREATMENT OF ESSENTIAL HTN

General

[Know treatment of HTN perfectly!]
Appropriate antihypertensive treatment decreases all hypertensive complications (stroke, LVH, CHF, renal failure), except coronary artery disease.

First: change bad habits. General lifestyle guidelines for preventing and controlling hypertension: Stop smoking. Lose weight if needed. Get regular aerobic activity. Moderate alcohol and Na^+ intake, maintain sufficient intake of K^+, magnesium, and calcium. Reduce intake of saturated fat and cholesterol.

If lifestyle changes are insufficient, initial drug therapy of uncomplicated Stage 1 essential HTN begins with the lowest doses of a thiazide diuretic. For Stage 2 hypertension, give a diuretic combined with a second agent. After 1–2 months, boost the dose, if necessary. If needed, 1 drug may be increased or changed for another drug. Try to give only once-per-day dosages for better compliance.

A different agent may be used as initial therapy if there is a "compelling" reason. These include: heart failure, post-MI, diabetes, chronic kidney disease, high cardiovascular risk, and recurrent stroke prevention (see Special Conditions below).

The Elderly

Hypertension is common in the elderly: 60–70% incidence! Elderly persons generally have isolated systolic hypertension, but diastolic HTN also occurs and you should treat both. The data now strongly supports treating isolated systolic hypertension in the elderly. The degree of systolic hypertension (good indicator) and the elevation of pulse pressure (even better!) are directly correlated with poor outcomes.

Treatment of HTN in the elderly begins with lifestyle changes. Especially decreasing weight and dietary salt. If drugs are needed:
• Start with low-dose thiazide diuretics.
• For isolated systolic HTN, use diuretics first, then long-acting calcium antagonists, unless there are other compelling indications (see next).

HTN TREATMENT FOR SPECIAL CONDITIONS

Special situations [Know!]:
• Angina pectoris: Beta-blockers and calcium antagonists are useful, but avoid short-acting calcium antagonists.
• Post-MI: Beta-blockers reduce recurrent MI; ACE inhibitors prevent subsequent heart failure and reduce other endpoints.
• LVH is a major risk factor for CV events. ACEI/ARBs, calcium-channel blockers, and sympatholytics cause regression of LVH! Diuretics have no effect. Of the direct vasodilators, hydralazine has no effect, while minoxidil increases LVH (avoid direct vasodilators). One study showed the best LVH regression with a diuretic and an ACE inhibitor. Note: The significance of decreasing LVH is uncertain.
• Patients with severe LVH have a small ventricular lumen and stiff ventricular muscle, causing a diastolic dysfunction (left ventricle ejection fraction is normal, but there is less to be ejected). Avoid preload reducers in these patients, and use diuretics with care.
• Heart failure: ACEI/ARBs alone or with diuretics, beta-blockers, aldosterone antagonists, or digoxin.
• Proteinuria > 1 g/24hr: Control BP to 130/85. Use ACEI/ARBs.
• Diabetes: ACEI/ARBs, alpha-blockers, calcium antagonists, and diuretics are preferred.
• Diabetic nephropathy: Use ACEI/ARBs as initial therapy
• Asthma: Avoid beta-blockers and alpha-beta blockers. ACEI/ARBs are safe in most.

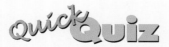

- Gout: Avoid diuretics (may induce or worsen hyperuricemia).
- Stroke: After an embolic/thrombotic stroke in a person with a history of HTN and vascular disease, do not treat HTN aggressively. The sclerotic vessels in the head need a higher perfusion pressure to function normally, and this is even truer after an ischemic stroke. If the blood pressure is very high, calcium-channel blockers are probably the best. Agents you should definitely avoid after an ischemic stroke are centrally acting agents (clonidine) and nitroprusside ("steals" blood flow from the brain).

HYPERTENSIVE CRISES

[Know!]

Hypertensive crises include any situation in which a rapid decrease in BP is required to limit end-organ damage. Signs of a hypertensive crisis with end-organ damage are very high blood pressure and: unstable angina, acute MI, encephalopathy, acute retinopathy, nephropathy, LV failure, and/or dissecting aneurysm.

There are 2 main syndromes caused by severe HTN that are clinical expressions of end-organ damage:

- Malignant HTN is severe HTN with papilledema or retinal hemorrhages or exudates. It also can cause malignant nephrosclerosis.
- Hypertensive encephalopathy is when there are signs of cerebral edema.

The many deleterious side effects of malignant HTN include deterioration of renal function, retinopathy from retinal artery spasm, and encephalopathy (from deranged autoregulation). The resulting intense hyperreninemic state may cause hypokalemia.

Treatment: Goal is to rapidly decrease diastolic BP to 100–105 mmHg within 2–6 hours—while minimizing the drop to ≤ 25%.

Generally IV agents are used but, if the patient is asymptomatic or there are no parenteral drugs available, you can use oral drugs. These drugs have a less controllable effect on blood pressure, and too rapid a drop in BP may cause ischemic problems like stroke or MI. Drugs used are loop diuretics, beta-blockers, alpha2-antagonists, and calcium antagonists. Avoid sublingual or oral (liquid) nifedipine and sublingual captopril.

In the setting of severe HTN with end-organ damage (malignant HTN, hypertensive encephalopathy, angina, dissection, etc.) always use IV agents: nitroprusside, labetalol, nicardipine (calcium-channel blocker), and fenoldopam (dopamine receptor agonist). IV agents give you better control but never drop blood pressure too fast!

SECONDARY HYPERTENSION

Renovascular HTN

The two main causes of renovascular hypertension are:
- renal artery atherosclerosis (often bilateral, mainly affecting men > 50 years old, especially diabetics; see Image 4-1) and
- fibromuscular dysplasia (also often bilateral, but mainly affecting women < 40 years old!)

Other causes of renovascular HTN are
- vasculitis, and
- scleroderma (1/2 of these patients have renovascular HTN!) and even Takayasu arteritis.

So consider renovascular HTN when you see moderate-to-severe HTN with onset in patients < 30 years old (fibromuscular), onset of HTN > 50 years old (atherosclerotic), and also with accelerated HTN.

Diagnosis: If renovascular HTN patients have an abdominal bruit caused by this condition, it is continuous (not just systolic). The combination of a continuous abdominal bruit and a low serum K$^+$ (hyperreninemic hyperaldosteronism—remember aldosterone facilitates active resorption of Na$^+$ and

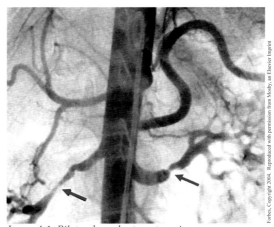

Image 4-1: Bilateral renal artery stenosis

secretion of K^+) in a hypertensive patient is strongly suggestive of renovascular HTN—especially if they have other risk factors (> 50 years old, diabetic).

Screen for renovascular HTN with captopril renogram or Doppler ultrasound.

Arteriography is the gold standard of diagnosis for renovascular HTN. Fibromuscular dysplasia shows up as a "string of beads" with multiple, little aneurysmal dilatations, whereas the atherosclerotic lesion is usually a single, unilateral, proximal stenosis with distal dilation. After a positive arteriography, you must do a renal vein renin test. If involved/uninvolved renin ratio > 1.5, then and only then is the lesion functionally significant!

Treatment: angioplasty. Beware: ACEI/ARBs decrease the blood pressure well, but also cause a decreased GFR in the involved kidney! This can cause prerenal azotemia and renal failure if the renal artery stenosis is bilateral! Having said that, particularly for scleroderma renal crises, ACEI/ARBs are the treatment of choice.

Primary Hyperaldosteronism

Aldosterone → Na^+ uptake from the distal tubule. Water follows the Na^+ and raised intravascular volume, thereby increasing blood pressure.

Suspect primary hyperaldosteronism in a person with hypokalemia of unknown etiology (not on diuretics). The person may or may not be hypertensive. There are two main causes of the primary form: adrenal adenomas (70%; Conn syndrome) and idiopathic bilateral adrenal hyperplasia (~ 25%); adrenal carcinoma is a rare cause. If the patient is not hypokalemic, don't even consider primary hyperaldosteronism.

Screening and diagnosis: Screening involves checking a stimulated plasma renin activity (PRA). If the stimulated PRA is low or undetectable, confirm the diagnosis by checking aldosterone level after salt and fluid loading: give 2 liters of normal saline IV over 3–4 hours. If the aldosterone level is not suppressed, the patient has primary hyperaldosteronism. Also, if the patient is already on an ACEI/ARB (ACEI or angiotensin II receptor blocker—see pg 4-15), draw renin and aldosterone levels to see if aldosterone is suppressed; if not, this also supports the diagnosis of 1° hyperaldosteronism. Do CT scan of the adrenals to look for adenoma.

Initial treatment of primary hyperaldosteronism is:
• salt and water restriction
• K^+-sparing diuretics: spironolactone, triamterene, amiloride
• +/- thiazide diuretic

Unilateral adrenal adenomas are surgically removed with excellent results, whereas patients with bilateral hyperplasia are managed with diuretics alone, because bilateral adrenalectomy resolves the HTN in only 33% of these patients.

Cushing Syndrome

Cushing syndrome is covered in the Endocrinology section.

Pheochromocytoma

Pheochromocytomas are very rare tumors arising from chromaffin tissue. 90% occur in the adrenal medulla. The rest are abdominal or thoracic. 10% are bilateral; 10% are malignant; and 10% are familial. Although commonly thought of with paroxysmal symptoms, 1/2 to 2/3 of patients have sustained HTN. Especially suspect this if the HTN is refractory to treatment. It is associated with MEN IIA and IIB.

Diagnosis: Screen with 24-hour urine for metanephrine, VMA, and catecholamines (the metanephrine test is least sensitive to interference from other meds). This screening is very specific and sensitive if it is collected while the patient is symptomatic, resting, and off meds.

To find the pheochromocytoma, CT the adrenals. If it is not found there, do arteriography or metaiodobenzylguanidine scintigraphy (norepinephrine analog, which concentrates in adrenals and pheos). Treat with surgery. Pre-op with phenoxybenzamine (alpha blockade) or labetalol to control blood pressure, then propranolol as needed for the tachycardia.

Pregnancy & HTN

There are two types of HTN that occur during pregnancy: chronic essential hypertension and pregnancy-induced hypertension.

If the HTN occurs before the third trimester, it is probably latent essential HTN, "brought out" by the pregnancy.

Pregnancy-induced HTN (PIH, preeclampsia) usually occurs in the 3rd trimester, and stops after delivery. When patients develop HTN, and proteinuria after the 20th week of gestation, usually in primigravidas, the diagnosis is PIH. Serum uric acid usually increases.

Severe PIH with elevated liver enzymes, low platelets, and microangiopathic hemolytic anemia is referred to as HELLP Syndrome.

Treatment of PIH is hospitalization, bedrest, and treatment of the HTN. Medications used are the tried-and-true methyldopa (drug of choice) and hydralazine. Labetalol and beta-blockers have been used. Limited experience with clonidine and calcium-channel blockers.

Avoid ACEI/ARBs (ACE inhibitors and angiotensin II receptor blockers—both teratogenic), and nitroprusside (cyanide poisoning) for PIH!

Avoid beta-blockers in early pregnancy (growth retardation).

Other Causes

Other important 2° causes of HTN that must be excluded include: birth control pills and coarctation of the aorta. Treatment of obesity, decreasing alcohol intake (to ≤ 2 drinks per day), and addressing a deficiency in calcium or potassium in the diet (no cause-effect proven) may normalize blood pressure in some patients with mild HTN.

notes

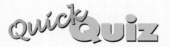

Quick Quiz

1) How do you confirm the diagnosis of primary hyperaldosteronism?

2) How do you screen for pheochromocytoma?

3) How does the trimester of occurrence relate to cause of hypertension in pregnancy (essential vs. PIH)?

4) What is the treatment for PIH?

5) What is the best first test to order in assessing acute renal failure?

6) What can you also order to differentiate between prerenal and acute GN?

7) What does the finding of a $FE_{Na} < 1\%$ and a normal urine sediment imply?

8) What are the causes of postrenal failure?

ACUTE RENAL FAILURE

OVERVIEW

We will now review the various causes of acute renal failure. Table 4-10 reinforces the important diagnostic points. There are 3 types of ARF, based on where the acute insult occurred:

I) Prerenal failure is usually due to an adaptive response to a problem causing decreased blood flow to the kidney.

II) Postrenal failure is simply due to blockage of the passage of urine.

III) Intrarenal or intrinsic renal failure is due to problems within the kidney. As we'll discuss, these often follow a similar sequence of clinical findings.

Rule out prerenal first, then postrenal, and then intrarenal.

A note on terminology. There is much overlap in the pathophysiology of these 3 classifications. For instance, there is blockage to urine flow with both the classic postrenal cases of outlet obstruction downstream of the kidney but also with cellular debris that accumulates in the tubules due to ATN—a classic intrarenal cause and intratubular obstruction. Also both postrenal and intrarenal causes typically have a secondary result of prerenal vasoconstriction.

Note: Oliguria is < 400 ml/d urine volume. Anuria is < 50 ml/d.

I. PRERENAL

Prerenal failure is always due to a real or "effective" decrease in renal blood flow:
- severe intravascular volume loss from volume depletion, blood loss, or (effectively) hypotension
- renal artery stenosis
- CHF and low output states
- drugs—especially diuretics (most common), NSAIDs, ACEI/ARBs, and (in transplant patients) interleukin-2, cyclosporine, and tacrolimus

If the cause is not obvious from the history, consider renal artery stenosis, especially if the onset was after surgery.

Note that renal emboli/thrombi can be considered prerenal (blocks renal blood flow) or intrarenal (usually affects small intrarenal vessels). In this discussion, these causes are placed under intrarenal causes.

NSAIDs are particularly likely to cause prerenal azotemia in patients whose renal function is compromised and, therefore, "prostaglandin-dependent" for normal function; e.g., Chronic Kidney Disease (CKD), edema states, and volume depletion.

If putting a patient on ACEI/ARB (ACE inhibitor or angiotensin II receptor blocker) causes prerenal azotemia, consider underlying atherosclerotic renal disease.

Patients with severe proteinuria (or with hypoalbuminemia of any cause: cirrhosis) have "effective" decreased renal blood flow and therefore are very susceptible to developing prerenal failure. Remember: With CHF, you have increased secretion of atrial natriuretic factor, but its effects in CHF are weak and are more than offset by the factors contributing to prerenal azotemia in CHF, including increased aldosterone and epinephrine.

Lab: BUN/Cr ratio is usually high. Urine is very concentrated with the urine osmolality often > 700. The urine Na^+ is < 20, indicating normal tubular function. Urine sediment is usually normal but can show granular or hyaline casts. The best, first test in assessing renal failure is the fractional excretion of Na^+ (FE_{Na})—this is very low (< 1%) in both prerenal azotemia and acute GN. To further differentiate between prerenal and acute GN, check urine sediment & protein. In general, if a patient has renal failure with a $FE_{Na} < 1\%$ and a normal urine sediment (or with just granular or hyaline casts), the patient has prerenal azotemia. See the equation for FE_{Na} on pg 4-1. Examine all of these patients for orthostatic hypotension.

II. POSTRENAL

Postrenal failure is usually due to bladder outlet obstruction (prostatic hypertrophy, stenosis, cancer). It can be caused by bilateral ureteral obstruction, but this is very rare. In postrenal failure, the BUN:Cr ratio is elevated (like in prerenal failure), because the urea diffuses back into the system. K^+ may be elevated due to associated Type 4 RTA (remember? Type 1 and 2 = low K^+, Type 4 = high). You see papillary necrosis (the papillae are just before the renal pelvis) in pyogenic kidneys with postrenal obstruction (and also in chronic analgesic abuse and sickle cell disease). You see sterile pyuria with WBC casts in the urine sediment; usually, the patient complains of renal colic and hematuria.

notes

III. INTRARENAL

Overview

Intrarenal failure—possible causes include:
- vascular problems
- acute tubular necrosis (ATN)
- intratubular obstruction
- glomerular damage (i.e., the acute glomerular nephritides—pg 4-22)
- acute interstitial nephritis (pg 4-30).

The most common vascular causes of intrarenal failure are renal artery emboli/ thrombosis/ stenosis, malignant HTN (rarer now), scleroderma, vasculitis, and eclampsia. Acute atheroembolic renal disease may have hypocomplementemia and, like vasculitis involving the kidneys, it can present with increased erythrocyte sedimentation rate (ESR), eosinophilia, and rash; but it does not have the RBC casts.

ATN and intratubular obstruction are discussed next and glomerular damage and AIN are discussed in their own sections following this section. Keep in mind that, although they are discussed in separate sections, AGN and AIN are intrarenal causes of ARF! (Want me to repeat that?)

ATN

Acute tubular necrosis is the most common cause of acute renal failure due to intrarenal causes (~ 75%!). Even so, you first must rule out other causes of acute renal failure. Although there is not always necrosis, tubular dysfunction is a hallmark of the disease. Overall, acute tubular necrosis is very serious; even with dialysis, 1/2 of surgical patients and 1/3 of medical patients die (usually because of multiple, other complicating factors). For those who improve, 90% do so within 3 weeks, 99% within 6 weeks.

ATN has various causes, the most common mechanism being a transient ischemic or toxic insult to the kidney. The most common cause is renal hypoperfusion, which is usually caused by surgery, but any other cause of shock can also cause it: trauma, burns, sepsis, cardiogenic.

ATN may also be caused by:
- myoglobinuria (rhabdomyolysis)
- hemoglobinuria
- heavy metals
- contrast dye
- drugs (aminoglycosides, amphotericin B, cisplatin, foscarnet)

Notes on drug-induced ATN:

Amphotericin B is especially likely to cause ATN at > 3 gm total dose. Amphotericin B has a direct nephrotoxic effect, and can cause a Type 1 or 2 RTA (see pg 4-9).

Aminoglycosides cause proximal tubule damage, resulting in a non-oliguric ATN! Aminoglycosides also cause hypomagnesemia.

Cisplatin is a common chemotherapy cause of ATN. Cisplatin also causes a magnesiuria and hypomagnesemia (this is its most asked about side effect).

Treatment of drug-induced ATN: Stop the drug and equilibrate input/output.

Urine lab and ATN: Urine is isoosmolar (osmolality < 400 but never < 300; Na^+ is > 20, FE_{Na} > 1%). Hallmark urine findings are large, muddy brown granular casts (nonspecific but very sensitive). Oliguric ATN usually resolves in 1–4 weeks. Note that oliguria is not required for the diagnosis of ATN; 25% of ATNs are the non-oliguric types (especially when caused by gentamicin)—this usually means less injury, not as high a BUN and creatinine, and a quicker recovery! If oliguric, ATN patients are very prone to becoming hyperkalemic.

Initial management of ATN includes treating the precipitating cause and any hyperkalemia. Match fluid input with output and encourage eating—which decreases catabolism! Stop drugs that may be the cause.

Table 4-10: Acute Renal Failure Lab Findings

ACUTE RENAL FAILURE	CAUSES	FeNa	URINE OSMOLALITY	URINE Na⁺	URINE SEDIMENT	SUSPECT IN PATIENT WITH...
PRERENAL	Volume depletion, NSAIDs, ACE inhib, Edema-forming states	< 1%	> 400 mOsm/L	< 20	Normal; or granular or hyaline casts	CHF, Chronic pain, Cirrhosis, Nephrotic syndrome, Bleeding
INTRARENAL (ATN) (so *after* acute GN, vascular diseases, AIN, and intratubular causes are ruled out)	ATN: Shock, Rhabdomyolysis, Contrast dye, Aminoglycosides, Pentamidine, Cisplatin	>>1%	300-350 mOsm/L	> 20	LARGE, muddy brown granular casts	Post contrast dye, Alcoholism, Severe hypokalemia
POSTRENAL	Prostatic hypertrophy, Cancer, Bilateral ureteral obstruction	Normal	Normal	Normal	Blood is common	Elderly male patients, Colicky pain

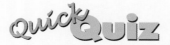

ATN Due to Rhabdomyolysis

Rhabdomyolysis is the end result of many mechanisms. The myoglobin released due to rhabdomyolysis can cause ATN if the urine is acidic and the patient is volume-depleted. Causes of rhabdomyolysis: muscle tissue trauma (2° comatose/OD with sustained muscle tissue compression or direct trauma to muscles), strenuous exercise, seizures, heat stroke, severe volume contraction, cocaine, hypophosphatemia, and severe hypokalemia.

Very elevated serum CPK level confirms rhabdomyolysis. If the serum CPK is unknown, suspect rhabdomyolysis by a high potassium, high phosphate, very high uric acid, low calcium, and a disproportionate increase in creatinine compared to the BUN.

Urine findings: As with other ATNs, muddy brown casts are common. The urine is heme-positive but without RBCs. The urine supernatant is often brown-to-pink.

Rhabdomyolysis-associated hypocalcemia results from 2 mechanisms: decreased production of 1,25-$(OH)_2D$ due to renal injury, and hyperphosphatemia due to both renal injury and tissue breakdown. The parathyroid hormone level is increased—in response to the low calcium.

Note: Although severe hypokalemia can cause rhabdomyolysis, the initial hypokalemia may not be evident at the time of diagnosis. Why is this? Because both the resultant muscle tissue breakdown and ATN tend to cause hyperkalemia. A similar problem can occur with rhabdomyolysis caused by hypophosphatemia.

Start treatment as soon as possible. There are 2 methods:
1) volume replacement with normal saline; and
2) forced diuresis and alkalinization of the urine.

Just as hypocalcemia is a complication of rhabdomyolysis, the patient is at risk for hypercalcemia during recovery. For this reason, do not treat hypocalcemia unless severe, or the patient is symptomatic.

Hemoglobinuria has similar urine findings as those seen in rhabdomyolysis. Hemoglobin can be released from severe intravascular hemolysis. It also can cause ATN—not due to toxicity, but rather mechanical obstruction. Treatment is the same as that for rhabdomyolysis (above).

Intratubular Obstruction

Intratubular obstruction is an intrarenal cause of ARF. It may be caused by urate nephropathy, oxalate depositions, hypercalcemia with intrarenal deposits, multiple myelomas, and certain drugs, especially methotrexate, indinavir, acyclovir, and sulfa antibiotics.

Cholesterol Atheroembolic Renal Disease—[Know!]—may be caused by aortic manipulation during surgery, vascular surgery, anticoagulants, and arterial catheterization of atherosclerotic patients. In this syndrome, there are showers of cholesterol emboli, which can affect the kidneys causing a "stepwise progression" of renal failure. The showers of emboli also can cause lesions and blue toes in the lower extremities (a skin biopsy of 1 of the lesions showing a cholesterol embolus is diagnostic).

So catheterization may cause 2 different renal problems. To differentiate: Contrast nephropathy (which occurs immediately) causes an acute renal failure, which then improves and has no skin findings.

A FEW PEARLS...

A few pearls for renal failure questions:
- If the patient is alcoholic, think rhabdomyolysis.
- If he has a prosthetic heart valve, think endocarditis with post-infectious GN.
- If he's being treated for CLL or lymphoma, think uric acid nephropathy.
- Drugs more often cause an interstitial nephritis than glomerular damage.

The history and physical generally give at least a good idea of the cause. There are some treatment points to know regarding ARF. Furosemide usually does not help preserve renal function in the presence of established ARF, especially if there is no increased urine output following its first use. Furosemide may be used, along with a saline bolus in early ARF, to try to convert it to a non-oliguric type, which is easier to manage. Low-dose dopamine is of use only in those patients with low blood pressure; often a fluid bolus is a more appropriate initial management. In general, sufficient volume loading is important for all types of ARF. Always treat the hyperkalemia.

MALIGNANCY-ASSOCIATED ARF

To summarize cancer and ARF: Malignancy-associated causes of ARF include lymphoma—when it infiltrates the kidney. Again, interleukin-2 causes severe prerenal azotemia in most patients! Both methotrexate and the uric acid formed from tumor lysis precipitate and obstruct the tubules. Cisplatin is directly nephrotoxic. Mitomycin C causes hemolytic uremic syndrome. Leukemia itself rarely affects kidney function. In

notes

patients with very high WBCs being treated with antimetabolites, do prophylaxis against uric acid nephropathy with allopurinol (probenecid is uricosuric and worsens nephropathy), maintain volume expansion, and alkalinize the urine. If you are unable to give allopurinol, then give furosemide with IV fluids and alkalinize the urine.

Remember: tumors also can cause obstruction.

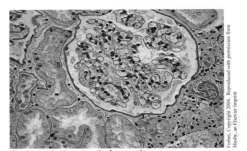

Image 4-2: A normal glomerulus

GLOMERULAR DISORDERS
OVERVIEW

Know this section well!

The glomerular apparatus: The glomerulus is merely a specialized capillary plexus. It is surrounded by the Bowman capsule. The capillary walls of the glomerulus are unique in that they filter blood—allowing an ultrafiltrate of the plasma to pass into the Bowman capsule—which in turn conducts the ultrafiltrate into the tubules for further processing. The wall of the glomerulus filters by means of 3 components:
1) the endothelial cells, then
2) glomerular basement membrane (GBM), and finally
3) slit pores between the epithelial cell foot processes.

Glomerular diseases are those that primarily affect the glomerular apparatus. They can be roughly divided into 2 classes, based on the mechanism of damage to the glomerulus:
1) Nephritic syndrome is an acute/subacute inflammatory process (also called "acute glomerulonephritis or AGN") that presents with hematuria, proteinuria and sometimes RBC casts.
2) Nephrotic syndrome presents primarily with heavy proteinuria and edema. Also urine fat ("oval fat bodies").

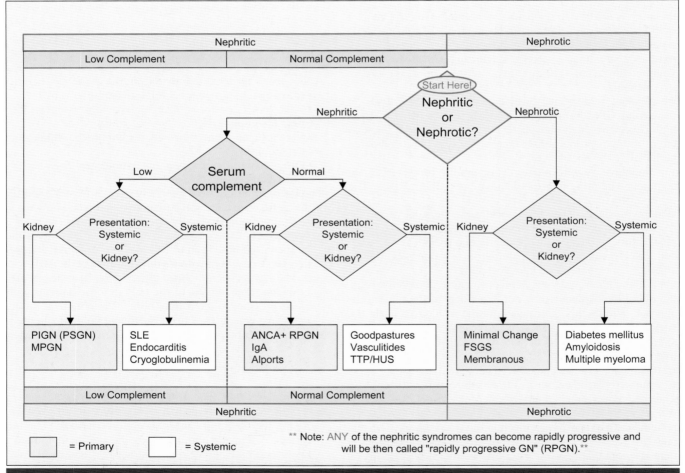

Figure 4-3 A Strategy for Workup of the Glomerular Disorders

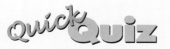

Quick Quiz

1) What type of kidney disease does heavy proteinuria and urine fat indicate?

2) What is the FE$_{Na}$ in all glomerulopathies?

3) Renal biopsy showing mesangial deposits confirms what diagnosis?

4) What are the differences between nephritic syndrome and nephrotic syndrome?

5) What does dysmorphic RBCs in urine sediment indicate?

6) Why do nephrotic patients become hypercoagulable?

7) Memorize Figure 4-3! Know this hot strategy cold!

8) What happens to complement levels in acute flares of Lupus nephritis?

Nephritic syndrome may "burn out" to nephrotic syndrome. The initial inflammatory and "proliferative" effects of nephritic syndrome are often reversible, but the later-occurring sclerosis is irreversible.

Glomerular disease causes are:
• idiopathic,
• antigen antibody (immune complex) trapped in the basement membrane or mesangium, or
• antibodies directed against the basement membrane.

The deposits in membranous GN and post-infectious GN are actually subepithelial, while they are mesangial in IgA nephropathy.

The FE$_{Na}$ is always < 1% in glomerulopathies. Acute glomerulonephritis is associated with sodium retention. This is due to intrarenal hemodynamic factors.

Achieve definitive diagnosis of all glomerulopathies with a renal biopsy. Light and electron microscopy reveal specific changes in the biopsy:

1) subepithelial deposits (membranous nephropathy and postinfectious GN),
2) subendothelial deposits (diffuse, proliferative, lupus nephritis and membranoproliferative GN), and
3) mesangial deposits (IgA nephropathy).

Refer to Figure 4-3, Figure 4-4, and Table 4-11 as you go through this section.

NEPHRITIC VS. NEPHROTIC

Nephritic urine indicates significant inflammation (itis) and glomerular damage. In the nephritic syndrome, there is variable proteinuria and "active" urine sediment; dysmorphic RBCs and WBCs; and casts of RBC, WBC, and granular material.

Casts always originate in the renal tubules, and you see RBC and WBC casts generally with nephritic syndrome (and interstitial nephritis)—and only rarely with nephrotic syndrome.

Granular casts are nonspecific; if you see only muddy brown granular casts on spun-down urine, ATN is more likely than GN (check the urine osmolarity—high in AGN and low in ATN!).

Classic causes of the nephritic syndrome include post-infectious GN, IgA nephropathy, and lupus nephritis. These will be discussed shortly.

Nephrotic urine reflects defects in the selectivity of the glomerular ultrafiltration barrier, even though there is little inflammation (think sclerotic). In nephrotic syndrome, there is typically heavy proteinuria and urine fat (free, fat droplets, oval fat bodies, fatty/waxy casts, and renal tubular cells with lipid droplets). The urine sediment is usually normal except for the fat.

Nephrotic range proteinuria is > 2.5–3.5 gm/d (or 40–50 mg/kg/d). Because of this protein loss, nephrotic patients tend to get hypoalbuminemia (with 2° edema), hypogammaglobulinemia (with a tendency for more infections, especially *H. influenzae* and *S. pneumoniae*), loss of thyroid and iron-binding globulins (so low total thyroxine and iron levels), and loss of antithrombin III (so they have a hypercoagulable state, and tend to get pulmonary emboli and renal vein thrombosis).

Nephrotic patients also have hyperlipidemia. When the albumin is very low, these patients often have severe peripheral edema, pleural effusions, and even ascites—yet they do not have pulmonary congestion/edema unless they have CHF. This is because the pulmonary interstitium loses albumin at the same rate as the blood, so there is not a big osmotic differential.

A strategy that helps classify the glomerular diseases is:

1) Is the urine Nephritic or Nephrotic?
2) Does the patient present with a Systemic disorder (by hx/physical) or primarily present with a Kidney disorder?
3) If the urine is nephritic, is the Complement Low or Normal?

While reading below, follow along in Figure 4-3. Know this flowchart! It gives structure to this otherwise quite confusing set of renal problems.

NEPHRITIC SYNDROMES

Complement

Flare-ups of "lupus nephritis" are always associated with hypocomplementemia; whereas with vasculitis, the hypocomplementemia is variable (usually normal, as shown in the chart). Complement is always low with PIGN and frequently low with MPGN (see next), which presents as kidney problems. It is also low with SLE, cryoglobulinemic GN, subacute bacterial endocarditis, shunt nephritis, and sometimes atheroembolic renal disease.

notes

RPGN

Okay, before we go into the method for classifying nephritic syndromes, let's review the one GN that any of the nephritic syndromes can evolve (devolve?) into—rapidly progressive glomerulonephritis (RPGN).

Again: **Any** of the nephritic syndromes is considered a RPGN *if* it becomes rapidly progressive with renal failure occurring within days to weeks. Hence, you can have RPGNs that have either high or low complement, or that present with systemic disease or primarily as a kidney disorder.

RPGN is mentioned in the footnote of Figure 4-3. There is one RPGN that always presents as rapidly progressive disease, and that is the ANCA+ RPGN. Therefore, it is given its own spot in this schema.

Always consider this if a patient presents with severe and progressive renal failure of recent onset. Once RPGN is diagnosed, you need to determine the disease process that is causing it.

In general, of the causes of RPGN, Goodpasture syndrome most often comes to mind, but more common causes are idiopathic, SLE, and vasculitis (one of the most frequent problems in Wegener granulomatosis and polyarteritis nodosa).

In Goodpasture syndrome, an anti-glomerular basement membrane antibody reacts and builds up linear deposits on the basement membrane (BM) of the kidney and lung, causing RPGN and pulmonary hemorrhage.

Pathologically, RPGN is grouped into 3 categories:
1) 45% are due to immune complex disease (post-infectious, lupus nephritis, IgA nephropathy, membranoproliferative, idiopathic).
2) 50% are due to pauci-immune disease (virtually no antibody deposition: microscopic polyangiitis, Wegener granulomatosis, Churg-Strauss: 80–90% ANCA-positive)
3) 5% are due to anti-GBM antibody disease (Goodpasture's or localized anti-GBM disease)

In RPGN, the urine has protein and RBC casts. There is glomerular capillary wall rupture, secondary to severe GBM damage, and > 50% of the glomeruli have crescents (quarter-moon-shaped structures that are a reflection of severe damage); it quickly progresses to end-stage renal failure. Inflammatory (cellular) crescents indicate disease that may respond to treatment, but fibrous crescents indicate irreversible disease.

Determining the cause of RPGN. Anti-GBM and ANCA. If there is a high titer of serum anti-GBM antibodies and the patient has pulmonary hemorrhage, the disease is Goodpasture syndrome. If there are anti-GBM antibodies and no pulmonary hemorrhage, it is just called "anti-GBM GN." As part of the initial evaluation, also check for anti-neutrophil cytoplasmic autoantibodies (ANCA).

If this is positive, consider 3 possibilities:
1) Wegener granulomatosis (has necrotizing pulmonary granulomas)
2) polyarteritis nodosa (has a systemic necrotizing arteritis)
3) idiopathic ANCA + crescentic GN (no systemic findings)
Most (> 90%) of Wegener patients are c-ANCA positive, while the latter two can have either p-ANCA or c-ANCA (more in the Rheumatology section).

If both the anti-GBM and ANCA are negative, consider the immune complex-related problems: lupus nephritis (check anti-ds-DNA antibodies), post-strep GN, and cryoglobulinemic GN (check cryoglobulin levels and complement—they should be low).

Treat RPGN with corticosteroids + cyclophosphamide or azathioprine. With SLE or ANCA+ vasculitis, always include the cyclophosphamide, because the relapse rate is decreased by a factor of 3! Treat cryoglobulinemic GN and Goodpasture's with plasmapheresis, followed by an alkylating agent.

Summary: 1) immune complex; 2) pauci-immune; 3) anti-GBM. Renal biopsy, steroids + cyclophosphamide. Know also that the lupus nephritis of SLE can produce almost any type of GN. Low complement occurs in cryoglobulinemic GN and lupus nephritis.

What are C3 and CH50? As discussed in the Allergy & Immunology section,

C3 is "used up" in both intrinsic and extrinsic complement reactions (and therefore, a marker for any complement reaction). Most diseases with immune complexes will show decreased C3 levels.

CH50 assay is a marker for the intrinsic pathway, so is normal when there is extrinsic activation.

Okay, now let's get back to the schema!

Nephritic with Low Complement— Primarily Kidney Presentation

> 1) Post-infectious GN (aka Post-Strep GN/PSGN)
> 2) Membranoproliferative GN-MPGN

1) Post-infectious **GN** (PIGN, diffuse endocapillary proliferative GN)—usually is thought of as due to Group A beta-hemolytic infection and called post-strep GN (PSGN), but actually, non-strep infections are the more common cause. Glomerular changes include diffuse cellular proliferation and hump-shaped subepithelial deposits (as can occur in membranous GN). It is usually caused by septicemia (endocarditis, pneumonia, etc.) or viruses, so think of this in a patient presenting with new-onset proteinuria, and RBC casts, and a history of any of these illnesses.

As with many of the acute GNs, this is caused by an antibody-antigen reaction, and here the source of the antigen is the infecting agent, causing granular deposits of IgG and C3 (from

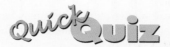

1) Which types of nephritis can acutely worsen into a RPGN?

2) What are the 3 categories of RPGN?

3) What are the first 2 antibody tests done in the workup of RPGN? Define the etiologies associated with the presence of each antibody.

4) What are the 3 ANCA+ causes of RPGN? Which one is almost always c-ANCA positive?

5) How long is the latency period for post-infectious GN?

6) Do post-streptococcal GN patients require treatment with antibiotics?

7) What disease is the usual cause of MPGN?

8) How can a C3 level help you differentiate poststreptococcal GN from MPGN?

$2°$ complement activation). It affects all the glomeruli and, on electron microscopy, the deposits show up as large subepithelial humps. This reaction causes hypocomplementemia with a decrease in serum level of C3 and a low CH_{50} assay for 6–8 weeks.

Post-streptococcal GN (PSGN—a subset of PIGNs): Certain nephritogenic strains of group A β–hemolytic strep causing a throat or skin (impetigo) infection will cause a GN, which occurs 1–6 weeks after the initial illness (average 10 days post-throat infections, 14 days after skin infections).

This "latency period" is a diagnostic key and is used in differentiating it from IgA nephropathy (next), in which the kidney GN immediately follows a viral illness.

Anti-streptococcal antibodies aid in the diagnosis of PSGN—check antistreptolysin O (ASO) titers—and/or anti-deoxyribonuclease B (anti-DNase B) titers. The ASO titers generally stay up for several weeks after a strep infection, the anti-DNase B titers for several months. [Hey! When else do you check these titers? Right!...in the workup of rheumatic fever.]

Post-infectious GN progresses to severe renal failure only if the infection persists. Therefore, always treat PIGN patients with antibiotics.

Most patients recover completely in 6–8 weeks. Progression is very rare, but is more common in adults than children.

Again: Treat the underlying infection with antibiotics (if bacterial), and there will be no progression to renal failure!!

Summary of PIGN: Reversible, treat the infection, epidemic, granular IgG and C3 deposits, low C3 and CH_{50} for about 6–8 weeks, usually no chronic renal failure.

2) Membranoproliferative GN.

Most cases of membranoproliferative GN (MPGN) are associated with HCV infection, which causes a mixed essential cryoglobulinemia in which C3, C4, and CH_{50} are low (classical complement activation), rheumatoid factor is very high, and cryoglobulins are present. MPGN frequently causes renal failure. Some cases remain idiopathic.

As the name suggests, "membranoproliferative" has both basement membrane (BM) changes and cell proliferation, like the mesangial proliferative GN (IgA nephropathy). The BM changes can cause nephrotic syndrome, whereas the cell proliferation is the nephritic component. This "double" GN also has BM changes in which the dense immune deposits make the BM look double-layered. What is not included in the name is that MPGN is also similar to the post-infectious (PIGN) in that there is often hypocomplementemia with a low C3 (in ~ 50%).

Note: The low C3 in post-infectious GN returns to normal after 2–3 months; whereas in patients with MPGN, it stays low indefinitely. This is useful: If you initially suspected PIGN and C3 stays low > 3 months, suspect MPGN instead, and get a renal biopsy!

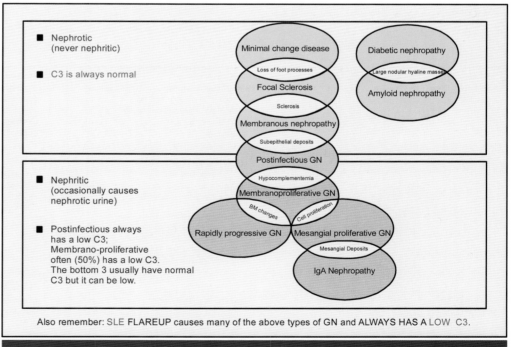

Also remember: SLE FLAREUP causes many of the above types of GN and ALWAYS HAS A LOW C3.

Figure 4-4: Comparison of the Glomerulonephropathies

notes

MPGN can present in different ways:
- with hematuria,
- with nephrotic-range proteinuria, or
- as a RPGN.

Treat children with prednisone and adults with ASA and dipyridamole. MPGN seems to be the only disease in which oral dipyridamole (di=double) is still considered useful! Treat MPGN associated with HCV with interferon.

Table 4-11: Summary Table of the Glomerulonephropathies

CLASSIFICATION/ COMPLEMENT Level		NAME	PRESENTATION	URINE	NOTES	TREATMENT
GLOMERULONEPHROPATHIES						
NEPHRITIC SYNDROME Primarily *Kidney* Presentation	Low	Postinfectious	1) Pt s/p hepatitis B presents with hematuria etc... 2) Pt s/p strep throat/ endocarditis/pneumonia...	"Nephritic" Hematuria with casts, proteinuria, and occ WBC/casts.	Complement level returns to normal after a short period.	If bacterial, treat the infection.
		Membranoproliferative	Usually with hematuria. Occasionally as RPGN or nephrotic syndrome.		Complement level stays low > 3 mo.	Children: steroids Adults: ASA and dipyridamole.
	Normal	ANCA+ RPGN	Idiopathic nephritic signs and symptoms.		Like other RPGNs	Corticosteroids with cyclophosphamide.
		IgA Nephropathy (Mesangial proliferative)	Young man c/o gross hematuria after exercise or with viral illness.		Commonest cause of acute GN. 50% of proteinurias go on to renal failure!	NO effective treatment!
		Alports	Nephritic syndrome with possible nerve deafness or congenital eye problems.		X-linked recessive	No specific treatment.
NEPHRITIC SYNDROME *Systemic* Presentation	Low		SLE, Subacute bacterial endocarditis, Cryoglobulinemia			Treat the cause.
	Normal		Goodpasture, various vasculitides. TTP/HUS.			Treat the cause.
NEPHRITIC SYNDROME RPGN		Rapidly progressive - see text for the many causes. Also = "crescentic" GN	SEVERE RENAL FAILURE OF RECENT ONSET!		Check ANCA and anti-GBM Ab.	Corticosteroids +/- cyclophosphamide or azathioprine. Treat RPGN with corticosteroids +/- cyclophosphamide (esp with SLE) or azathioprine. Cryoglobulinemic GN is treated with plasmapheresis and then an alkylating agent.
NEPHROTIC SYNDROME Primarily *Kidney* Presentation		Minimal Change Disease	Child with nephrotic syndrome. Adult with nephrotic syndrome and no pathologic changes seen in the renal biopsy on light microscopy.	"Nephrotic" Heavy Proteinuria (> 2.5-3.5 gm/d) and FAT droplets.	2nd commonest primary cause of nephrotic syndrome in adults (20%). Commonest cause in children. Renal failure is rare.	Children: steroids - excellent response. Adults have a much slower response. Also may try cyclophosphamide or cyclosporin if no response to steroids in an adult.
		Focal Sclerosis	Nephrotic syndrome and IV drug abuser, has AIDS, hematologic malignancies, chronic vesicoureteral reflux, or is obese.		3rd commonest primary cause of nephrotic syndrome in adults (15%).	40% go into remission with same tx as minimal change disease; 60% go on to end stage renal disease!
		Membraneous nephropathy	Rheumatoid arthritis patient on gold or penicillamine presents with nephrotic synd. If no drug history, rule out solid tumor.		Commonest primary cause of nephrotic syndrome in adults (30-40%). Susceptible to renal vein thrombosis.	Relatively benign. Corticosteroid alone not effective. Steroid plus a cytotoxic agent (cyclophosphamide or chlorambucil) is better.
NEPHROTIC SYNDROME *Systemic* Presentation		Diabetic nephropathy	Diabetic with nephrotic-range proteinuria		Commonest secondary cause of nephrotic syndrome.	Low protein diet and HTN control
		Amyloidosis and multiple myeloma	"Skin popper" drug addict.			

notes

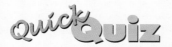

1) When does hematuria usually occur in a patient with IgA nephropathy?

2) For patients with IgA nephropathy, what tests give a good indication of prognosis?

3) Know Table 4-11! ☺

4) Which 6 diseases cause nephritic syndrome with normal complement levels? Which of these have a primarily kidney presentation? Which have a primarily systemic presentation?

Summary: double name, double BM, low C3, C4, and CH$_{50}$ (like PIGN), steroids for kids, ASA and dipyridamole for adults.

Nephritic with Low Complement— Systemic Presentation

1) Systemic Lupus Erythematosus (SLE). Know also that the lupus nephritis of SLE can produce almost any type of nephritic (or nephrotic) glomerular disease.
2) Endocarditis
3) Cryoglobulinemia

Nephritic with Normal Complement— Primarily Kidney Presentation

1) ANCA+ Rapidly Progressive Glomerulonephritis (RPGN)
2) IgA Nephropathy
3) Alport syndrome

1) ANCA+ RPGNs. These are the ANCA+ RPGNs with no systemic findings (so not Wegener's or PAN). These are discussed earlier under RPGNs (pg 4-24).

2) IgA nephropathy (mesangial proliferative GN; aka Berger disease). Nephritic. Worldwide, IgA nephropathy is the most common GN (>25%).

IgA nephropathy is also known as "mesangial proliferative"— i.e., there is mesangial hypercellularity with small crescents when severe.

The antibody-antigen reaction in this disease is reflected by immune complex deposition of IgA and C3 in the mesangial matrix and skin. Although C3 is deposited, there are usually normal serum complement levels; only occasionally are they low. IgA nephropathy is more progressive in patients with proteinuria and relatively innocuous in those with hematuria only.

IgA nephropathy has a wide range of presentations, from gross hematuria immediately following a URI, to microscopic hematuria with proteinuria and progressive disease. The hema-

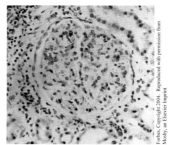

Image 4-3: IgA Nephropathy (Mesangial proliferative GN)

turia seen in IgA nephropathy commonly occurs either during a viral illness or just after exercise. It is more common in Asians and males.

Schönlein-Henoch purpura (HSP). While this causes IgA in the mesangium, it is a vasculitis (see below).

Occasionally, the culprit is IgM, and this is simply called IgM nephropathy. Test questions usually present a man (maybe Asian) who has gross hematuria either after exercising or during a viral illness.

Prognosis for IgA nephropathy is tied to serum creatinine, blood pressure, and amount of proteinuria. Prognosis is good if these values are normal, but it is much worse if any of these are abnormally elevated. 50% of these patients with proteinuria have inexorably progressive renal disease. There is no consensus on treatment, although ACEI/ARBs (ACE inhibitors and angiotensin II receptor blockers) and fish oils appear to help.

Summary: IgM and IgA (MesAngial), Berger, no effective treatment.

3) Alport syndrome is a hereditary (usually X-linked) syndrome with chronic glomerulonephritis and sometimes nerve deafness and congenital eye problems (discussed on pg 4-33).

Nephritic with Normal Complement— Systemic Presentation

1) Goodpasture syndrome
2) Vasculitides
3) TTP/HUS

1) Goodpasture syndrome is discussed earlier under RPGN (see beginning of "Nephritic Syndromes").

2) Vasculitides: Wegener granulomatosis and polyarteritis nodosa (PAN) are also discussed under RPGN. Schönlein-Henoch purpura (HSP) is seen mostly in children. It has identical kidney findings, but also affects the skin, GI tract, and joints. Patients may have abdominal and joint pains, erythema, urticaria, and of course purpura and hematuria.

3) TTP and hemolytic uremic syndrome are discussed in the Hematology section.

notes

NEPHROTIC SYNDROME

Note

The following glomerulopathies cause a nephrotic urine (i.e., proteinuria without active/nephritic sediment).

Nephrotic—Primarily Kidney Presentation

> 1) Minimal Change Disease
> 2) Focal and Segmental Glomerulosclerosis (FSGS)
> 3) Membranous Nephropathy

1) Minimal change disease is the most common cause (90%!) of nephrotic syndrome in children < 10 years old ("minimal change in small change"). It also causes 15–20% of the nephrotic syndromes in adults.

Although there is heavy proteinuria, there is usually no hematuria. It is usually idiopathic, but can be caused by NSAIDs and is associated with Hodgkin disease. Often, in accordance with the name, there is no change in histology on light microscopy, but electron microscopy shows loss of the epithelial cell foot processes. Urine sediment may show "Maltese crosses" under polarized light.

Minimal change disease has a good response to steroids (first choice), cyclophosphamide, or cyclosporine. Minimal change disease has the best prognosis of the nephrotic syndromes. Children with nephrotic syndrome are usually treated empirically with corticosteroids. Perform a renal biopsy if the expected response to steroids does not occur.

Summary: nephrotic range proteinuria, children, NSAIDs, loss of foot processes, Maltese crosses, steroids, best prognosis.

2) Focal and segmental glomerulosclerosis (FSGS)—Typically idiopathic, FSGS is similar to minimal change disease in that there is diffuse foot process loss; some cases of focal sclerosis may actually be a more severe form of minimal change disease. These patients have kidney sclerosis, but only in segments of the glomeruli, especially the juxtamedullary glomeruli. FSGS has become the most common cause of idiopathic nephrotic syndrome in African Americans. Especially consider FSGS if the nephrotic patient is between 15 and 30 years old and is hypertensive. Also consider FSGS if there is a history of: HIV+, obesity, sickle cell disease, hematologic malignancies, or chronic vesicoureteral reflux.

These patients have slowly progressive renal failure. Those not responding to treatment require dialysis within ~ 5 to 10 years.

Treat FSGS with long-term steroids to get patients into remission. Prognosis for FSGS is worse than that for minimal change disease. 40% go into partial or complete remission

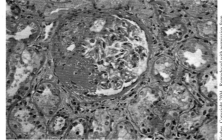

Image 4-4: FSGS

with corticosteroids; 60% go on to end-stage renal disease.

Summary: nephrotic range proteinuria, loss of foot processes and focal sclerosis, African-Americans, young hypertensive, AIDS, obesity. Treat with long-term steroids.

3) Membranous nephropathy is a common idiopathic cause of non-diabetic nephrotic disease in adults, but there may be underlying causes, which include [Know]:
- Chronic infections, such as malaria, HBV (especially), HCV, and syphilis;
- Several drugs—especially gold, penicillamine, and NSAIDs;
- Also, a small percentage of patients presenting with membranous nephropathy may have underlying solid tumors. These tumors are almost always clinically obvious, with appropriate age-standard cancer screening.
- SLE can also cause this type (remember, it can cause most types of glomerulopathy!).

It is an indolent process and presents the same as focal sclerosis (later), but the renal biopsy shows involvement of all the glomeruli. Membranous nephropathy, like postinfectious GN, may have subepithelial IgG and C3 deposits—most of the deposits are intramembranous. Membranous nephropathy has hypocomplementemia only if it is due to a SLE flare-up.

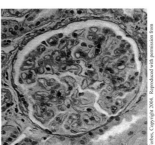

Image 4-5: Membraneous nephropathy

Women have a much better prognosis than men. Overall, ~ 30% slowly progress to renal failure.

Treatment is controversial. Mild cases frequently have spontaneous remission. Use corticosteroids plus a cytotoxic agent (cyclophosphamide or chlorambucil) in severe, progressive cases.

Summary: nephrotic range proteinuria, HBV. Gold, penicillamine, solid tumors, SLE. Worse prognosis in men. If severe, treat with corticosteroids plus a cytotoxic agent.

Nephrotic—Systemic Presentation

> 1) Diabetes mellitus
> 2) Amyloidosis and Multiple Myeloma
> 3) SLE

1) Diabetic nephropathy is the most common cause of nephrotic syndrome in adults. The nephropathy develops in 30% of Type I diabetics! The microvascular retinopathy usually follows decline in renal function.

The first, easily measurable change in renal function is microalbuminuria. Microalbuminuria represents amount of albumin too small to detect on routine dipstick (30–300 mg/24 hr). It can be detected by measuring the random urine protein/creatinine ratio. > 30 mg/24 hr represents a positive test. Test all diabetics yearly for microalbuminuria and, if posi-

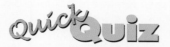

Quick Quiz

1) "Maltese crosses" seen in urine sediment is indicative of what abnormality? (No—not *Babesia*, this is nephrology, not ID).

2) Children with nephrotic syndrome usually have what type of abnormality? Does it usually respond to steroids in children? in Adults?

3) FSGS is found in what patient groups?

4) Patients with solid tumors and nephrotic syndrome usually have what type of renal disease?

5) When will membranous nephropathy also have hypo-complementemia?

6) A diabetic patient has rapid deterioration of renal function. Is this likely due to diabetic nephropathy?

7) What factors decrease the rate of progression of diabetic nephropathy?

8) Congo-red staining of the renal biopsy from a patient with amyloidosis and light chain nephropathy shows what findings?

9) NSAIDs cause what types of renal disease?

---

tive, treat with an ACEI or ARB (see pg 4-15), even if normotensive.

Renal biopsy, though not usually necessary for diagnosis, shows diffuse and then nodular changes in the glomerulus. Onset of the nephropathy is followed by progressive decrease of renal function, and dialysis or transplant is required within 5–7 years after the onset of proteinuria. It is unlikely to occur within 5 years or > 35 years of onset of the diabetes. If a diabetic has rapid decrease in renal function, such as over several months, it is almost certainly not due to diabetic nephropathy alone; look for other causes of renal failure.

Excellent control of HTN, glucose levels, and the use of an ACEI/ARB slow the rate of deterioration. Low-protein diet was thought to slow the rate of deterioration, but this has come under question since the results of the NIH study of MDRD (Modification of Diet in Renal Disease)—so the jury is still out on this.

Tight blood glucose control has also been shown to slow the progression of diabetic nephropathy (DCCT and other trials).

As renal function decreases, insulin requirements decrease (2° to decreased metabolism by the kidneys)! As mentioned before, diabetic nephropathy often causes decreased renin. This results in a hyporeninemic hypoaldosteronism and Type 4 RTA—pg 4-9.

2) Amyloidosis may cause light chain nephropathy. Light chain nephropathy causes light microscopic changes, similar to those in diabetic nephropathy. So, if you see a renal biopsy with very large hyaline-appearing nodular masses in the glomerulus, think of diabetic or light chain nephropathy. To differentiate: Congo red stain of amyloid characteristically has a unique "apple-green birefringence" when viewed with the polarizing microscope.

There are various causes and various biochemical types of amyloidosis. The "AL" type is the primary cause of amyloidosis, and is also the type that is associated with multiple myeloma (MM). The AL type is caused by a plasma cell clone line producing partially degraded kappa or lambda fragments.

This is not the "light chain disease" commonly caused by MM, even though both MM and amyloidosis can cause a nephrotic renal disease, and both have some form of light chains. The MM light chain deposits do not have the unique staining with Congo red dye. The "AA" type is seen in amyloidosis due to chronic inflammation, such as rheumatoid arthritis and familial Mediterranean fever (FMF).

Rarely, amyloid nephropathy may result from the chronic skin infections that result from "skin-popping" by drug addicts.

Use colchicine in the treatment of FMF to prevent amyloidosis.

Drugs and Nephrotic Syndrome

Drugs that cause nephrotic syndrome include NSAIDs, oral gold, penicillamine, trimethadione, and captopril (rarely). What other renal disease do NSAIDs cause? Right! Papillary necrosis (see postrenal failure, pg 4-19—which is also caused by analgesic abuse).

Treatment of Nephrotic Syndrome

General principles: Treatment of nephrotic syndrome depends on the underlying disease. Control of glomerular pressure is vital in any glomerulopathy; increased intraglomerular pressure hastens disease progression. ACEI/ARBs are best in decreasing intraglomerular pressure and are usually used along with a low-protein diet, which also decreases intraglomerular pressure. Use diuretics prn, but be careful—patients with nephrotic syndrome usually have difficulty maintaining intravascular volume, and the salt restriction and diuretics can precipitate prerenal failure. Note that corticosteroids +/- cytotoxics are used in most nephrotic syndromes—except those caused by amyloid and diabetes. Anticoagulation is used if there is a significant risk of thrombosis (especially membranous nephropathy).

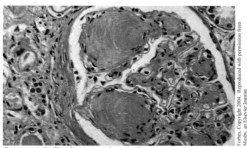
Image 4-6: Diabetic nephropathy

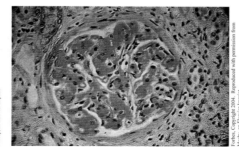
Image 4-7: Renal amyloidosis

notes

Again [Know]: Hypocomplementemia always occurs in post-infectious and frequently in membranoproliferative GN. There is also hypocomplementemia in cryoglobulinemic GN and in flare-ups of SLE (which cause any type of glomerulo-pathy). Other diseases with low complement levels are subacute bacterial endocarditis, shunt nephritis, and sometimes atheroembolic renal disease.

The following usually have normal complement (i.e., only occasionally low): RPGN, IgA (mesangial proliferative) GN, Wegener granulomatosis, and Goodpasture syndrome.

Hypocomplementemia never occurs in the nephrotic syndromes: minimal change disease, FSGS, membranous nephropathy, diabetic nephropathy, or amyloid nephropathy.

And again [Know]: Nephritic (= active; = casts of WBCs, RBCs, and granules) urine sediment is usually seen in IgA nephropathy (mesangial proliferative), early post-infectious, membranoproliferative, SLE, and RPGN. Remember that nephritic sediment does not exclude nephrosis, although this usually does not occur early on in nephritic-type nephropathies. Nephritic sediment is never seen in the nephrotic syndromes: minimal change, focal sclerosis, membranous nephropathy, diabetic nephropathy, and amyloid nephropathy. Note that these are the same diseases in which hypocomplementemia never occurs!

And again [Know! ☺]: Urine sediment in renal disease.
- Prerenal failure: "benign" U/A, occasionally granular casts and hyaline casts.
- Postrenal: frequently is "benign," may have blood; WBC casts if due to papillary necrosis.
- Intrarenal: ATN: large, muddy brown granular casts.

Glomerulopathies: nephritic (hematuria with RBC casts, and sometimes pyuria with WBC casts) and nephrotic (fat bodies). AIN (see next): eosinophils, RBCs, WBCs, and WBC casts.

And again: Use steroids in most nephrotic syndromes—except those caused by amyloidosis and diabetes. Also use steroids in RPGN and when MPGN affects children.

TUBULAR AND INTERSTITIAL DISEASES

ACUTE INTERSTITIAL NEPHRITIS

Tubular and interstitial diseases have only slight proteinuria (< 1–1.5 gm/d), and they may cause renal tubular acidosis (RTA).

Acute (or allergic) interstitial nephritis (AIN) is a drug-induced hypersensitivity problem and often presents with eosinophilia.

The urine sediment in AIN is different from GN in that it does not have the heavy albuminuria, RBC casts, or fat bodies. With AIN, the urine sediment may have eosinophils, RBCs, WBCs, and WBC casts. They also have beta-2 microalbuminuria.

The drugs that most commonly cause AIN include antibiotics, NSAIDs, cimetidine, thiazides, phenytoin, and allopurinol.

The most common antibiotic culprits are the beta-lactams—especially methicillin, TMP/SMX, cephalosporins, and rifampin. Fluoroquinolones are another cause. Antibiotics cause a classic triad of fever, rash, and eosinophilia. It is an idiosyncratic response to the antibiotic and is not related to the amount of antibiotic or the antibiotic's duration of use.

NSAID-induced AIN is different in that the NSAIDs are typically ingested for months before symptoms occur. The rash, fever, and eosinophilia may not occur. Contrary to all other types of AIN, with NSAID-induced AIN, there is usually nephrotic range proteinuria with minimal change glomerular changes. Acute interstitial nephritis also can be caused by sarcoidosis, SLE, infection (pyelonephritis) and transplant rejection.

CHRONIC INTERSTITIAL NEPHRITIS

Chronic interstitial nephritis is caused by:
- renal outlet obstruction
- drugs: chronic analgesic abuse, cisplatin, cyclosporine
- heavy metals (especially lead and cadmium)
- Sjögren disease
- sickle cell disease
- multiple myeloma

Regarding the above: Chronic interstitial nephritis is associated with papillary necrosis from chronic analgesic abuse—especially mixtures containing more than one analgesic—and NSAIDs. To get it, a person needs to ingest > 6 pounds of drugs!!! Cumulative. It is also caused by heavy metals, especially lead (with associated hyperuricemia and gout) and cadmium. Note that penicillamine causes glomerular disease—not interstitial nephritis!

Consider chronic interstitial nephritis in the patient with a history of frequent pain who presents with proteinuria and an elevated creatinine. Check for lead toxicity with EDTA. Any time a patient is spilling glucose in the urine, yet has **normal serum glucose**, think tubulointerstitial disease (other examples are Type 2 RTA [pg 4-9] and pregnancy!) Remember that NSAIDs can cause either an acute (within days) or chronic interstitial nephritis. The most impressive (and asked about) aspect of this NSAID-induced acute nephritis is the high proteinuria—usually in the nephrotic range.

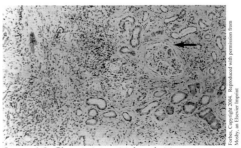

Forbes, Copyright 2004. Reproduced with permission from Mosby, an Elsevier Imprint

Image 4-8: Chronic interstitial nephritis

notes

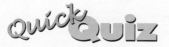

Remember: If there is a question with renal dysfunction and high proteinuria, think of nephrotic syndrome or NSAID-induced nephritis. If light proteinuria and active sediment, then consider both nephritic syndrome (especially IgA nephropathy) and tubulointerstitial disease (nephritis), as discussed above.

OTHER DRUG-INDUCED NEPHROPATHIES

Drug-induced Acute Tubular Necrosis (ATN) is discussed on pg 4-20.

NSAID effects on the kidney: Decreased GFR is the most common renal effect of NSAIDs. Decreasing renal blood flow (by blocking the prostaglandins that vasodilate) may cause prerenal azotemia. So, especially avoid NSAIDs in patients with decreased renal function or low flow/volume states. NSAIDs also decrease renin release, exacerbating the tendency for hyperkalemia in a patient with hyporeninemic hypoaldosteronism. If a person has a stimulated renin-angiotensin system, as during a prerenal stress, such as CHF or volume contraction, they are especially susceptible to hemodynamic compromise due to NSAIDs. As mentioned above, NSAIDs can also cause an acute or a chronic interstitial nephritis—usually with nephrotic range proteinuria.

Review of drug-abuse renal problems. Chronic IV drug abusers are at risk for several types of kidney problems.

1) Acute bacterial endocarditis causes either focal or progressive glomerulonephritis by immune complex deposition in the kidney.

2) It can also damage the kidney from septic embolization, resulting in renal infarct and hematuria.

3) A chronically progressive focal sclerosis is occasionally seen in IV drug abusers.

4) After the accessible veins are gone, IV drug abusers often resort to "skin-popping" and then develop chronic subcutaneous infections, which cause amyloidosis and amyloid nephropathy.

CHRONIC KIDNEY DISEASE
OVERVIEW

The current practice guidelines have changed chronic renal failure (CRF) to chronic kidney disease (CKD).

Chronic kidney disease (CKD) is defined as:
- kidney damage > 3 months, with or without decreased GFR, with either pathological abnormalities or markers of kidney damage, or
- a GFR < 60 ml/min > 3 months, with or without kidney damage.

There are 2 elements to consider:
1) the original disease/insult, and
2) after 3/4 of nephrons are gone, the remaining ones that are forced to take over for the non-functioning ones. The secondary hyperperfusion and hypertrophy result in further loss of renal function.

The most common cause of CKD is non-insulin-dependent diabetic nephropathy. It is important to rule out reversible causes, including chronic CHF and obstructive uropathy. Stop any NSAIDs, aminoglycosides, and beta-lactam antibiotics. Treat any hypercalciuria, hyperphosphatemia, HTN, or UTI.

If a patient presents with a microcytic anemia, CKD, and gout, what must you think of? Answer: lead nephropathy.

Systemic effects: CKD causes HTN, a normochromic, normocytic anemia (from decreased erythropoietin), and salt retention with volume overload, all of which can precipitate CHF. It may cause "restless leg syndrome" or a peripheral sensory neuropathy.

Patients with end-stage renal disease (ESRD) have 2 types of bone disorders: 1) a high bone-turnover disorder, and 2) a low bone-turnover disorder:
1) The high bone-turnover state is called osteitis fibrosa cystica, and is characterized by a high PTH with secondary increased osteoclast and osteoblast activity.
2) A low bone-turnover state is characterized initially by osteomalacia, and later by adynamic osteodystrophy. This was caused by aluminum toxicity when it was used as a phosphate binder to decrease hyperphosphatemia in these patients. Control hyperphosphatemia with Ca^{++}-containing binders ($CaCO_3$ or Ca acetate), or sevelamer (Renagel®) and lanthanum (Fosrenol®)—to keep the Ca x P product < 55.

CKD also can cause decreased glucose tolerance, decreased gonadal hormone production (with impotence or amenorrhea/infertility), and a low T_3 with a normal TSH.

The uremia itself may cause uremic pericardial and pleural effusions, hemorrhagic pericarditis, anorexia, and an increased anion gap metabolic acidosis. Uremia does not cause any liver dysfunction.

notes

GOUT IN CKD

Gout can occur in CKD. An exacerbation can still be treated with colchicine or NSAIDs, although you must monitor kidney function of patients on NSAIDs. Allopurinol decreases the production of uric acid, and chronic usage is often necessary. Probenecid usually works by increasing renal excretion of uric acid. In CKD, of course, it is not effective and contraindicated.

TREATMENT OF CKD

Progression of CKD is slowed by ACEI/ARBs (ACE inhibitors or angiotensin II receptor blockers) and possibly by reduced protein intake. ACEIs and ARBs are known to decrease intraglomerular pressure but, in addition, more recent data suggest that angiotensin II turns on TNF-β, which stimulates fibrosis, and this also may be suppressed by ACEIs/ARBs.

The normochromic normocytic anemia in CKD responds dramatically to recombinant erythropoietin. Before starting treatment, first ensure there are plenty of iron stores on board (i.e., Fe saturation and ferritin levels are normal).

DIALYSIS

Dialysis—When to start? Answer: When the CKD patient has advancing uremia. This usually means any uremic symptoms in a patient with a CrCl < 15 ml/min.

Starting at a particular BUN or creatinine value is of no proven benefit. A forearm AV fistula lasts the longest, but should be created several months before dialysis; otherwise, a prosthetic graft is needed. Refer patients when serum creatinine is ~ 4.0 mg/dl.

The most common cause of death in dialysis patients is cardiovascular problems. Next is infection. The most common cause of admission is thrombosis/infection of the vascular access.

Dialysis patients have anemia, high triglycerides, and a low HDL. They usually have a metabolic acidosis just before and a respiratory alkalosis just after dialysis.

Another dialysis-associated problem is metabolic bone disease—which can be either secondary hyperparathyroidism or a vitamin D-resistant osteomalacia (low bone-turnover renal osteodystrophy). Note that dialysis does not cause loss of either vitamin D or calcium!

Maintaining adequate nutrition in these patients is one of the key factors in reducing morbidity and mortality. Vitamin supplements are indicated, especially folate and iron.

Continuous Ambulatory Peritoneal Dialysis (CAPD). With CAPD, you do not need an AV fistula or an expensive machine, and it causes less strain on the heart.

The patient infuses 2–3L of hypertonic dextrose solution into the peritoneal cavity (subsequently drained by gravity) 4–6 (or more) times per day.

For CAPD, the main complication is peritonitis, usually caused by Gram-positive skin flora (usually *S. epidermidis* or *S. aureus*), and next most commonly, Gram-negative organisms. Outpatient treatment of the peritonitis is usually successful with intraperitoneal antibiotics! Other CAPD problems include high protein loss (12 gm/d!!) and loss of water-soluble vitamins (especially folic acid).

Decreased renal function increases the half-lives of many drugs. Vancomycin is the extreme example; it can be given once every 7 days if the GFR < 10% of normal!

RENAL TRANSPLANT

If there is renal function deterioration in the first week after transplant:
- check cyclosporine or tacrolimus levels,
- do a renal ultrasound to rule out outlet obstruction and then, if levels okay and ultrasound (–),
- do a renal biopsy.

Cyclosporine decreases T-cell proliferation (but not function!) without affecting the bone marrow. Side effects of cyclosporine include tremors, nephro/hepato/CNS toxicity, and hypertension. Dose-related nephrotoxicity causes the most problems. Also, like phenytoin, it hypertrophies the gums. Cyclosporine and tacrolimus are metabolized by the cytochrome P-450 system. Blood levels of cyclosporine are increased by erythromycin, ketoconazole, and diltiazem—and decreased by phenytoin, carbamazepine, rifampin, and phenobarbital.

Tacrolimus has the same mode of action and similar profile as cyclosporine, but it is also diabetogenic.

Azathioprine has completely different side effects from cyclosporine. It does affect the bone marrow. The most significant side effect is leukopenia. Allopurinol increases serum levels of azathioprine. Not used much anymore with transplants.

Mycophenolate mofetil (MMF, CellCept®) is a newer agent now used more frequently than azathioprine. It has a similar profile, but its main side effects are GI with less BM suppression.

Note: On the board exam, you will probably be asked about either drug interactions or the side effects of cyclosporine, tacrolimus, MMF, and maybe azathioprine (although azathioprine has fallen out of favor). Know also that any type of long-term immunosuppressive therapy is associated with neoplasia.

Urinary tract infections, pneumonia, and sepsis are the most common infections after kidney transplant, but the main cause of death is cardiovascular-related. CMV infection is a common problem (see the Infectious Disease section). Prophylactic acyclovir prevents herpes and prophylactic SMP-TMX prevents PCP. Renal transplant patients are also more

notes

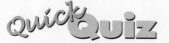

1) What measures slow the progression of CKD?

2) How may normocytic normochromic anemia in CKD be treated?

3) When is dialysis initiated in a CKD patient?

4) What drugs increase cyclosporine levels? Decrease?

5) What can reverse the late manifestations of small-vessel calcification and motor neuropathy?

6) What 3 organs or systems does Alport's affect?

7) Which type of chronic renal failure will present with a normal urinalysis with no proteinuria?

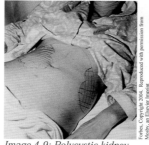
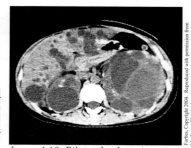

Image 4-9: Polycystic kidney disease

Image 4-10: Bilateral polycystic kidneys

likely to get post-transfusion hepatitis, aseptic necrosis of femoral heads, and cataracts.

Renal diseases that may recur after transplant include rapidly progressive GN, mesangial (IgA, Berger's), membranoproliferative GN, and idiopathic focal/segmental sclerosis. Post-infectious GN and interstitial nephritis do not recur.

Both dialysis and renal transplant reverse the platelet dysfunction, renal osteodystrophy, and sensory and cognitive dysfunction. Only transplant can reverse the late manifestations of small vessel calcification and motor neuropathy.

HEREDITARY KIDNEY DISEASES

ALPORT

Alport syndrome = Hereditary nephritis (also discussed under normal complement nephritic syndromes on pg 4-27). Alport syndrome can be either X-linked or autosomal dominant (AD) with variable expression. Men are affected more seriously than women.

Alport syndrome results from a connective tissue defect (of Type IV collagen), which affects the basement membrane (the same target as the Goodpasture's anti-GBM antigens!), cochlea (occasional, associated deafness), and the lens. The female X-linked carriers have microscopic hematuria only. The affected males have renal failure before age 50.

Consider Alport syndrome in any patient with persistent microscopic hematuria (onset at birth) that worsens after an infection (i.e., include this in the differential diagnosis of post-infectious GN and IgA nephropathy). Also, especially consider Alport syndrome in a woman with microscopic hematuria when there is a family history of males dying of kidney problems. Diagnose with a kidney biopsy in both men and women.

POLYCYSTIC KIDNEY

Polycystic kidney disease (AD) is the most common genetic disease of the kidney. It is usually associated with a mutation on the short arm of chromosome 16. There is a locus near the defective gene that, if found, suggests a tendency for the disease. Patients get cysts of the kidneys, liver, and pancreas, as well as associated recurrent hematuria.

Onset of polycystic kidney disease occurs at ~ age 20. Progressive renal failure and HTN are the norm. The liver cysts cause hepatomegaly but rarely liver dysfunction. Cerebral aneurysms occur in a very small percent (1–5%); they occasionally cause problems, but you don't need to screen unless the patient is symptomatic or there is a family history of cerebral aneurysms.

The diagnosis is usually established when polycystic kidneys are identified by imaging (U/S or CT) during evaluation for hematuria.

For kidney infections, use the lipid-soluble antibiotics such as quinolones, trimethoprim, erythromycin, chloramphenicol, tetracycline, and clindamycin—because they penetrate better.

MEDULLARY DISEASE

There are 2 main inherited medullary kidney diseases:
- Medullary sponge disease (diagnosed by IVP), which is rarely clinically significant but associated with high PTH, hypercalciuria, and renal stone disease
- Medullary cystic disease, which can cause renal failure. Medullary cystic disease is one of the few types of chronic renal failure in which there usually is a normal urinalysis without proteinuria.

notes

PREGNANCY AND RENAL DISEASE

Suspect pregnancy-induced hypertension (PIH, or preeclampsia) in a patient with new-onset HTN, proteinuria, and rapid weight gain with edema after 20-weeks gestation. Patients may have diffuse vasospasm, a low-grade DIC with associated decreased platelets, and a decreased antithrombin III (good diagnostic test). Severe cases may develop HELLP syndrome (hemolytic anemia, elevated liver function tests, low platelets). Treatment: delivery of the infant. More on pg 4-18.

SLE with lupus nephritis. If the disease has been in remission, there is a 90% chance of a successful pregnancy. If SLE flares up during pregnancy, however, 25% of the fetuses die, usually from the lupus anticoagulant antibody causing thrombotic events. Screen all pregnant lupus patients for lupus anticoagulant (spontaneous abortion) and SSB antibodies (neonatal heart block).

Pregnancy and CKD. If the creatinine is < 2 and the patient with CKD is not hypertensive, there is not an increased risk of abortion or malformation, and there is no increase in the rate of progression of the renal disease. There is an increased risk of preeclampsia.

As renal failure progresses, a woman's chance of pregnancy decreases. Dialysis patients rarely become pregnant. In stable renal transplant patients, the outcome of pregnancy is usually great!

RENAL CYSTS

Renal cysts are very common: 50% of people > 50 years old have them. They are considered benign if the patient is asymptomatic and if, by ultrasound, they are simple cysts; i.e., well-defined margins, no echoes, and dense (compressed) surrounding tissues. Otherwise, surgical exploration is indicated to rule out cancer. Also see polycystic kidney disease above.

RENAL STONES

Renal stones. Most (2/3) renal stones are calcium stones (calcium phosphate or calcium oxalate); the other 1/3 are either struvite or uric acid. Struvite is a phosphate stone with a mixture of cations: calcium/ ammonium/ magnesium phosphate.

Workup following initial stone passage usually includes:
- chemical analysis of the stone
- calcium level (to rule out a hyperparathyroidism problem)
- electrolytes (to rule out Type 1 distal RTA)
- U/A with C+S
- renal imaging (spiral CT is the imaging of choice; rarely use IVP)

For recurrent stones, check urine for the following: volume, cystine, calcium, Na, urea, uric acid, citrate, and creatinine. If there are signs of acute ureteral obstruction with a concurrent kidney infection, the patient must be hospitalized, because sepsis and papillary necrosis may result.

There are several factors that inhibit or promote stone formation. Citrate is the major inhibitor of calcium stones, but magnesium and pyrophosphate are also inhibitors. Concentrated urine and/or excretion of excessive amounts of stone-forming products cause precipitation and stone formation. Finally, certain products may act as a nidus for stone formation.

Calcium stone inducers: hypercalciuria, uric acid, hypocitraturia, hyperoxaluria, and medullary sponge disease. Citrate chelates calcium, thereby preventing stones. Acidosis (RTA etc.) causes hypocitraturia (< 250 mg/24 hr—Know this value!) and also leaches calcium from the bones, resulting in hypercalciuria. Although the calcium stones are usually a combination, they are often grouped into calcium phosphate and calcium oxalate stones.

Hypercalciuria can be caused by hypervitaminosis D, distal (Type 1) RTA, sarcoidosis, and hyperparathyroidism. 1/2 of the patients have idiopathic hypercalciuria, which is usually due to increased calcium absorption from the gut, caused by an increased renal production of $1,25\text{-}(OH)_2\ D3$, but it can also be due to a renal calcium leak.

Calcium phosphate stones are more common in patients with distal (Type 1) RTA because of the hypercalciuria just mentioned, with 1° hyperparathyroidism, and in those on acetazolamide. The distal RTA causes an alkaline urine that increases precipitation of $CaPO_4$ and the associated metabolic acidosis predisposes stone formation, because it buffers calcium out of the bones.

High urinary oxalate is the most important factor in calcium oxalate stone formation. Vitamin C and ethylene glycol are oxalate precursors and, theoretically, can cause stones if taken in large amounts (ethylene glycol will kill you first!) Steatorrhea also causes oxaluria; free fatty acids in the bowel chelates the calcium, allowing the oxalate to be absorbed and then excreted in the urine. Uricosuria is a predisposing factor for oxalate stones, because the uric acid crystal is similar to calcium oxalate and can act as a nidus for stone formation.

Treat calcium stones by pushing fluids, giving thiazide diuretics (decrease urinary calcium), decreasing dietary protein and

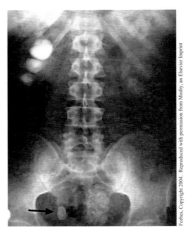

Image 4-11: Several urinary calculi

notes

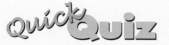
sodium (!), giving potassium citrate prn, and treating high uric acid. Note: Do not decrease calcium intake; this only increases oxaluria!

Struvite (calcium/ammonium/magnesium-phosphate) stones grow quickly and often cause staghorn calculi. Think infection when you see staghorn calculi. The ammonium needed to make these stones occurs only when urease breaks down the urea. This urease is produced by *Proteus*, *Pseudomonas*, yeast, and Staph (PPYS, "piss"), but especially the *Proteus* group. Treatment consists of removal of the stones/calculi, acidification of the urine (this is the only other stone, besides calcium phosphate, made more likely by alkaline urine), and antibiotics. If all of the stones or calculi cannot be surgically removed, patients require indefinite antibiotic treatment.

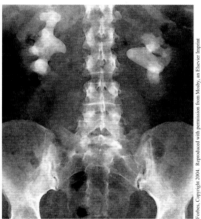

Image 4-12: Bilateral staghorn calculi

Forbes, Copyright 2004. Reproduced with permission from Mosby, an Elsevier Imprint

Cystine stones are due to cystinuria. Cystine is undersaturated in the normal urine, but patients who are homozygous for cystinuria (autosomal recessive [AR]) excrete large amounts. Look for clear hexagonal crystals in the urine. Cystine is very insoluble. It is usually best to treat by increasing fluids and by alkalinizing the urine—to keep urine cystine concentration normal! Penicillamine forms soluble complexes with cystine but is not well tolerated. Heterozygotes do not form stones.

Uric acid stones are usually seen in patients who chronically excrete acidic urine. You also see them in those who have high serum uric acid. Myeloproliferative syndromes, chemotherapy, and Lesch-Nyhan syndrome can cause such hyperuricosuria that there is stone formation even at normal urine

pH. Treat with allopurinol +/- urinary alkalinization. Give allopurinol before treatment of high cellular tumors. Avoid urinary alkalinization if there is also hypercalciuria.

Treatment options for acute ureteral obstruction include 1) allow passage, 2) remove via cystoscope, 3) U/S—either by percutaneous ultrasonic lithotripsy or by extracorporeal shock-wave lithotripsy (ESWL). ESWL use never became widespread and is now fading.

Again note [Know]: Urinary alkalinization is done for all types, except struvite and calcium phosphate. Also remember the difference between cystine and citrate: Cystine is an amino acid that precipitates into stones, while citrate chelates calcium in the urine, thereby preventing stones.

KIDNEY-ASSOCIATED ANEMIAS

CKD causes a decrease in the erythropoietin, which results in a normocytic normochromic anemia responsive to recombinant erythropoietin. Start patients with anemia due to CKD on erythropoietin therapy after assuring they have adequate iron stores. The target Hgb in these patients is 11–12 mg/dl.

Goodpasture syndrome can cause an anemia (microcytic/hypochromic) from chronic blood loss in the lungs.

Malignant hypertension may cause a microangiopathic hemolytic anemia and thrombocytopenia.

Sickle cell disease results in anemia and causes kidney disease.

APPENDIX A

Derivation of the Henderson equation.

The Henderson equation is derived from the bicarbonate buffer equation:

$$HCO_3^- + H^+ \leftrightarrows H_2CO_3 \leftrightarrows H_2O + CO_2 \qquad (eq\ 1)$$

H_2CO_3 is carbonic acid. HCO_3^- is bicarbonate. CO_2 is carbon dioxide. In the serum, these 3 molecules exist in equilibrium with one another.

From the law of mass action is derived the dissociation constant for carbonic acid K_{Ai}:

$K_{Ai} = (H^+ \times HCO_3^-)/H_2CO_3$; and since CO_2 is in equilibrium with H_2CO_3, this equilibrium constant is added to K_{Ai}, and we get:

$$K_A = (H^+ \times HCO_3^-)/ CO_2 = H^+ \times (HCO_3^-/ CO_2)$$

Taking logarithms:

$$\log K_A = \log H^+ + \log (HCO_3^-/ CO_2)$$

so:

$$-\log H^+ = -\log K_A + \log (HCO_3^-/ CO_2)$$

Noting that dissolved CO_2 is a function of the partial pressure of CO_2 in blood, $CO_2 = .03\ P_aCO_2$; and that $pH = \log [1/H^+] = -\log [H^+]$, we get the Henderson-Hasselbalch equation:

$$pH = pK + \log (HCO_3^-/.03P_aCO_2) \qquad (eq\ 2)$$

notes

The following material is to assist you in integrating the information you have just reviewed in this section. These are purposely NOT Board-style questions since they are meant to cover a lot of material in minimal space. MedStudy does have Board-style Q&A products separately available in book and software formats.

SINGLE BEST ANSWER

1) A. Eosinophiluria.
   B. Benign transient proteinuria.
   C. Proteinuria.
   D. Microalbuminuria.
   E. Benign orthostatic proteinuria.

1. Best indicator of underlying renal pathology.
2. Proteinuria while standing.
3. Drug-induced nephritis.
4. Proteinuria only after exercise.
5. Best indicator of early renal pathology.

[1 (C) 2 (E) 3 (A) 4 (B) 5 (D)]

2)

	pH	P_aCO_2	P_aO_2	HCO_3^-
A.	7.56	30	80	30
B.	7.37	60	55	33
C.	7.43	46	86	36
D.	7.40	60	60	36
E.	7.38	35	70	28

1. Compensated respiratory acidosis with an additional metabolic alkalosis.
2. Compensated metabolic acidosis with an additional metabolic alkalosis.
3. Respiratory alkalosis plus a mixed metabolic acidosis and alkalosis.
4. Compensated metabolic alkalosis.
5. Compensated respiratory acidosis with an additional metabolic alkalosis.

[1(B) 2 (E. The pH is 7.38 so you know the basic problem is an acidosis. The P_aCO_2 is low so it is compensating for a metabolic acidosis. The HCO_3^- is higher than expected so there is also a metabolic alkalosis.) 3 (A. The decrease in P_aCO_2 accounts for at most 0.8 of the increase in pH, so we already know there must be a metabolic alkalosis in addition to the respiratory alkalosis. The bicarb reflects both a compensation for the respiratory alkalosis and the additional metabolic alkalosis. If it were higher, it would more likely be acute [uncompensated] respiratory alkalosis plus a metabolic alkalosis.) 4 (C) 5 (D. The HCO_3^- is slightly higher than would be expected. The giveaway is that the pH is 7.4. This looks like an overcompensation, which doesn't happen! Think of this in a dehydrated COPD patient [contraction alkalosis].)]

3) Hyponatremia:
   A. Isotonic hyponatremia.
   B. Hypertonic hyponatremia.
   C. Low volume hypotonic hyponatremia.
   D. Normal volume hypotonic hyponatremia.
   E. High volume hypotonic hyponatremia.

1. Hyperglycemia.
2. High K^+.
3. SIADH.
4. Congestive heart failure.
5. Low K^+.
6. Mannitol.
7. Hyperlipidemia.
8. Hypoalbuminemia.
9. Multiple myeloma.

[1 (B) 2 (C. Low Na^+ and high K^+ are the hallmark of adrenal insufficiency in which there is Na^+ and water loss (more Na^+ than water). Other causes of low-volume hypotonic hyponatremia are diuretics and GI losses—vomiting and diarrhea.) 3 (D. This can also be caused by diuretics if there is sufficient free water replacement.) 4 (E. These patients typically present with edema.) 5 (D. The most common cause of hypotonic hyponatremia is diuretics and, if the patient is isovolemic, there is also usually an associated hypokalemia.) 6 (B) 7 (A) 8 (E. As with CHF, these patients present with edema.) 9 (A)]

4) Hypernatremia:
   A. Low-volume hypernatremia.
   B. Normal-volume hypernatremia.
   C. High-volume hypernatremia.

1. Diabetes insipidus.
2. Dehydration.
3. Primary hyperaldosteronism.

[All hypernatremic states are hyperosmolar. 1 (B) Central vs. nephrogenic DI is differentiated with the water restriction test. 2 (A) 3 (C)]

5) Kidney physiology:
   A. Proximal tubule.
   B. Descending loop of Henle.
   C. Ascending loop of Henle.
   D. Distal tubule.
   E. Collecting duct.

1. Site of action of spironolactone.
2. Site of action of acetazolamide (Diamox®).
3. Site of action of antidiuretic hormone.
4. 90% of bicarbonate is resorbed here.
5. K^+ and H^+ excreted via the electrical gradient here.
6. Site of action of furosemide.
7. Free water only removed.
8. Most calcium is resorbed here.
9. 25% of NaCl is actively resorbed here.

[1 (D. Spironolactone is an aldosterone antagonist. Aldosterone facilitates the active resorption of Na⁺ in the distal tubule.) 2 (A) 3 (E) 4 (A) 5 (D) 6 (C. Also bumetanide and ethacrynic acid are active here in the lower, thin ascending loop of Henle. Thiazides are active in the upper, thick ascending loop of Henle.) 7 (B) 8 (A) 9 (C)]

6) Renal tubular acidosis:
    A. Type 1 RTA.
    B. Type 2 RTA.
    C. Type 4 RTA.
    D. All of the above.
    E. None of the above.

1. Normal anion gap.
2. Bicarbonate wasting.
3. Defect in H⁺ secretion.
4. Defect in the Na⁺/K⁺/H⁺ exchange mechanism in the distal tubule.
5. Proximal RTA.
6. Mimics the effect of acetazolamide.
7. Mimics spironolactone.
8. Treated with furosemide.
9. Heavy metal poisoning.
10. Diabetic nephropathy.
11. Hypercalcuria.
12. Multiple myeloma.
13. Renal stones.
14. Always low [K⁺].
15. High [K⁺].
16. Low to normal [K⁺].

[1 (D) 2 (B) 3 (A) 4 (C) 5 (B) 6 (B) 7 (C) 8 (C) 9 (B) 10 (C) 11 (A) 12 (B) 13 (A) 14 (A) 15 (C) 16 (B)]

7) A. Hyperkalemia.
    B. Hypokalemia.
    C. Hypercalcemia.
    D. Hypocalcemia.
    E. Hypermagnesemia.
    F. Hypomagnesemia.
    G. Hyperphosphatemia.
    H. Hypophosphatemia.

1. Past history of neck irradiation.
2. Diabetic nephropathy.
3. This is a side effect of gentamicin but not cisplatin.
4. Volume contraction.
5. This is commonly seen in alcoholics.
6. Acutely caused by acute tubular necrosis.
7. May be seen in renal failure patients with a history of constipation.
8. If severe, treatment is IV calcium, followed by insulin plus glucose.
9. This is a side effect of both gentamicin and cisplatin.
10. Occasionally seen after the treatment of eclampsia.
11. Often treated with furosemide.
12. Often treated with thiazide diuretics.

[1 (C. These patients have post-irradiation primary hyperparathyroidism.) 2 (A) 3 (B) 4 (A) 5 (H) 6 (G. This may also be caused acutely by tumor lysis.) 7 (E. This occurs when renal failure patients treat their constipation with Mg-containing laxatives.) 8 (A) 9 (F) 10 (E) 11 (C. Also remember that furosemide can cause hypocalcemia.) 12 (D. Also note that thiazide diuretics can cause hypercalcemia.)]

8) Secondary causes of hypertension:
    A. Renovascular hypertension.
    B. Primary hyperaldosteronism.
    C. Pheochromocytoma.
    D. Pregnancy-induced hypertension.

1. ACE inhibitors and nitroprusside should not be used.
2. Low K⁺.
3. Atherosclerosis or fibromuscular dysplasia.
4. Clonidine decreases diagnostic test results while MAO inhibitors and labetalol may cause falsely elevated results.

[1 (D. ACE inhibitors are teratogenic and nitroprusside may cause cyanide poisoning.) 2 (B. Remember that primary hyperaldosteronism has 2 main causes: adrenal adenomas and idiopathic bilateral adrenal hyperplasia. It is screened for by checking a stimulated PRA.) 3 (A. Also scleroderma.) 4 (C)]

9) A. Atenolol (Tenormin®).
    B. Metoprolol (Lopressor®).
    C. Nadolol (Corgard®).
    D. Pindolol (Visken®).
    E. Propranolol (Inderal®).
    F. Timolol (Blocadren®).

1. Beta-1 agonist activity, somewhat lipid-soluble.
2. Very lipid soluble, no beta-1 selectivity.
3. Lipid soluble and strong beta-1 selectivity.
4. Not lipid soluble, not beta-1 selective.
5. Not lipid soluble and strong beta-1 selectivity.

[1 (D) 2 (E) 3 (B) 4 (C) 5 (A)]

10) Beta-blockers
    A. Lipid-soluble.
    B. Not lipid-soluble.
    C. Not applicable.

1. Atenolol (Tenormin®) and nadolol (Corgard®).
2. Shorter half-life with increased first-pass effect.
3. Beta-1 agonist activity.
4. Decreased central effect.

[1 (B) 2 (A) 3 (C) 4 (B) The way to remember these is: only atenolol (Tenormin®) and nadolol (Corgard®) are not lipid-soluble, and only atenolol (Tenormin®) and metoprolol (Lopressor®) are beta-1 selective antagonists—at low doses. Only pindolol (Visken®) has any beta-1 agonist activity—which has nothing to do with lipid solubility.]

11) Acute renal failure: Classification and associated lab findings.
   A. Prerenal.
   B. Postrenal.
   C. Intrarenal: glomerulonephritis.
   D. Intrarenal: acute interstitial nephritis.
   E. Intrarenal: vascular.
   F. Intrarenal: ATN.

[Abbreviations key:
Fractional excretion of Na = FE_{Na}
Urine osmolality = $Urine_{Osm}$
Urine Na = $Urine_{Na}$
Urine sediment = $Urine_{Sed}$]

1. $Urine_{Sed}$ = RBCs but no casts. All other findings are normal.
2. $Urine_{Sed}$ = many granular casts, FE_{Na} = .5%, $Urine_{Osm}$, = 800, $Urine_{Na}$ = 10.
3. $Urine_{Sed}$ = large brown granular casts, FE_{Na} = 5.0%, $Urine_{Na}$ = 50.
4. $Urine_{Sed}$ = RBCs, WBCs, WBC casts, and eosinophils.
5. $Urine_{Sed}$ = RBC casts and WBC casts; FE_{Na} is 0.7%.

[1 (B) 2 (A) 3 (F. The key word is "large"—nonspecific granular casts are usually small. The urine is also hypo-osmolal [< 400 mOsm/L] in ATN.) 4 (D. The key word is "eosinophils" in acute interstitial nephritis [AIN].) 5 (C)]

12) A. Fusion of foot processes.
   B. Sclerosis.
   C. Subepithelial deposits.
   D. Hypocomplementemia (Low C3).
   E. Basement membrane changes.
   F. Cell proliferation.
   G. Large hyaline masses.

1. Membranous nephropathy and post-infectious GN.
2. Membranoproliferative GN and rapidly progressive GN.
3. Minimal change disease and focal sclerosis.
4. Post-infectious GN and membranoproliferative GN.
5. Diabetic and amyloid nephropathies.
6. Focal sclerosis and membranous nephropathy.
7. Membranoproliferative GN and mesangial proliferative GN.

[1 (C) 2 (E) 3 (A) 4 (D) 5 (G) 6 (B) 7 (F. There's no easy way to learn this. Just memorize the diagram in the section.]

13) A. Minimal change disease.
   B. Focal sclerosis.
   C. Membranous nephropathy.
   D. Postinfectious GN.
   E. Membranoproliferative GN.
   F. Rapidly progressive GN.
   G. Mesangial proliferative GN.
   H. Diabetic nephropathy.
   I. Amyloid nephropathy.

1. Most common cause of nondiabetic nephrotic syndrome in adults.
2. Basement membrane changes and cell proliferation.
3. Think of this type of GN when the patient has Wegener granulomatosis, Goodpasture syndrome, or SLE and severe renal failure of acute onset.
4. Consider this with GN associated with hypocomplementemia lasting > 3 months.
5. Think of this in drug abusers who "skin-pop."
6. Think of this as a probable cause of a nephrotic GN in IV drug abusers.
7. GN in a patient who had hepatitis B.
8. Most common cause of nephrotic range proteinuria in adults.
9. Elevated IgA.
10. This GN is associated with solid tumors.
11. This is a form of Henoch-Schönlein purpura.
12. This crescentic GN is what other types of GN may evolve into.
13. Main cause of GN in children.

[1 (C) 2 (E) 3 (F) 4 (E) 5 (I. "AA" type amyloidosis—and nephropathy—occurs in patients with chronic skin infections.) 6 (B. It also occurs in persons with AIDS, hematologic malignancies, chronic vesicoureteral reflux, and obesity.) 7 (D) 8 (H) 9 (G. This is also called IgA nephropathy.) 10 (C) 11 (G) 12 (F) 13 (A)]

14) A. Acute interstitial nephritis.
   B. Chronic interstitial nephritis.
   C. Both.
   D. Neither.

1. Drug-induced hypersensitivity reaction with eosinophilia.
2. Trimethoprim sulfamethoxazole.
3. Multiple myeloma.
4. Penicillamine.
5. Papillary necrosis from chronic analgesic abuse.
6. Sjögren syndrome.
7. Lead-caused interstitial nephritis.
8. Associated with NSAID use.

[1(A) 2 (A. Other antibiotics associated with acute interstitial nephritis are methicillin, rifampin, fluoroquinolones.) 3 (B) 4 (D. Penicillamine causes glomerular disease—not tubulointerstitial disease.) 5 (B) 6 (B) 7 (B) 8 (C)]

15) Post-transplant medications
   A. Cyclosporine.
   B. Azathioprine.
   C. Both.
   D. Neither.

Which drugs are associated with the following?
1. Bone marrow suppression with leukopenia.
2. Decreased T-cell function.
3. Blood levels are increased by erythromycin.
4. Nephrotoxicity, hepatotoxicity, and neurotoxicity.
5. Blood levels are decreased by both phenytoin and phenobarbital.
6. Neoplasia.
7. Hypertension and tremors.

[1 (B) 2 (D) 3 (A) 4 (A) 5(A) 6 (C) 7 (A)
Cyclosporine decreases T-cell proliferation (but not function!) without affecting the bone marrow. Side effects of cyclosporine include tremors, nephro-/hepato-/CNS toxicity, and hypertension. Also, like phenytoin, it hypertrophies the gums. Cyclosporine is metabolized by the cytochrome P-450 system. Blood level of cyclosporine is increased by erythromycin, ketoconazole, and diltiazem. They are decreased by phenytoin, carbamazepine, rifampin, and phenobarbital.
Azathioprine has completely different side effects from cyclosporine. It does affect the bone marrow. The most significant side effect is leukopenia. Allopurinol increases serum levels of azathioprine. All long-term immunosuppressants cause neoplasias.

16) Hereditary kidney diseases:
    A. Alport syndrome (Hereditary nephritis).
    B. Polycystic kidney disease.
    C. Medullary disease.

1. Associated deafness.
2. Occasionally associated with cerebral aneurysms.
3. Most common genetic disease of the kidney.
4. Mutation of the short arm of chromosome 16.
5. Affects the liver and pancreas also.
6. Affects the basement membrane, cochlea, and lens.
7. Normal urinary sediment.
8. Persistent microscopic hematuria, which worsens after infections.
9. Gross hematuria.

[1 (A) 2 (B. 1–5% incidence in patients with polycystic kidney disease.) 3 (B) 4 (B) 5 (B) 6 (A) 7 (C) 8 (A) 9 (B)]

17) Renal stones:
    A. Calcium stones.
    B. Uric acid stones.
    C. Struvite stones.
    D. Cystine stones.

1. Staghorn calculi.
2. Seen in patients who excrete acidic urine.
3. Associated with *Proteus*, *Pseudomonas*, yeast, and staphylococcal infections.
4. Hexagonal crystals.
5. Seen in patients with Type 1 RTA.
6. Associated with myeloproliferative syndromes.
7. Citrate is a major inhibitor of this type of stone.
8. Associated with steatorrhea.
9. Treatment includes thiazide diuretics.
10. May require antibiotic treatment for an indefinite period.
11. Elevated uric acid, hyperoxaluria, and hypocitraturia induce these types of stones.

[1 (C) 2 (B) 3 (C. Especially *Proteus*.) 4 (D. Cystine stones occur only in patients who are homozygous for cystinuria.) 5 (A) 6 (B) 7 (A) 8 (A. Calcium oxalate stones.) 9 (A. Thiazide diuretics decrease calcium excretion.) 10 (C) 11 (A). Also remember that treatment for cystine and uric acid stones can include alkalinizing the urine, whereas treatment for struvite stones can include acidifying the urine.]

CASE HISTORIES

18) A 24-year-old AIDS patient being treated for PCP is found to have a serum creatinine of 1.8. A week before, the serum creatinine was 0.8. Which of the following is true?

    A. The patient most likely has AIDS nephropathy.
    B. The cause of the increased creatinine is probably trimethoprim.
    C. A kidney biopsy is indicated.
    D. The patient probably has *Pneumocystis*-related post-infectious nephritis.
    E. The BUN/Cr ratio is likely to be > 20.

[B. Trimethoprim, along with probenecid and cimetidine, decrease the tubular secretion of creatinine.]

19) A 34-year-old patient with no significant past medical history arrives with altered mental status. The only abnormality on the electrolytes is a low HCO_3^-. What is the working diagnosis?
    A. Methanol poisoning.
    B. Heroin overdose.
    C. High anion gap metabolic acidosis.
    D. Severe volume depletion.
    E. Normal anion gap metabolic acidosis.

[C. Although methanol poisoning is a cause of high anion gap acidosis, calling it that now would be jumping to conclusions.]

20) A 65-year-old smoker presents with hyponatremia. He has no edema and is not on diuretics. He has no significant medical history. There are no orthostatic changes in blood pressure. All other routine lab tests are normal.
    A. This patient almost certainly has lung cancer.
    B. This patient is probably hyperglycemic.
    C. Slow diuresis is indicated.
    D. Multiple myeloma is a possible cause of these lab values.
    E. Intravenous hypertonic saline infusion is indicated.

[D. Because the BUN and glucose are normal (assumably—which you can do in these and board questions because they are not given as abnormal), this patient has a hypotonic hyponatremia. The other information given indicates he has normal-volume status. The most common cause of this condition is SIADH. Increased ADH may be due to lung cancer or MM (Okay, this is one of those trick questions.) Lung cancer is still the most likely cause in this setting, but answer option (A) says he almost certainly has lung cancer—which is false—and (D) says it is a possible cause—which it most certainly is.]

21a) A previously healthy, normal-weighted 33-year-old man from Brazil visits you complaining of malaise and dyspnea on exertion. On physical exam BP is 165/110, and he is noted to have bibasilar inspiratory wet rales and 3+ pedal edema. CBC and electrolytes are normal. Urine analysis: 4+ protein and moderate fatty casts. Serum albumin is 2.2 g/dL.

Which of the following is not important in the patient's history:
A. Recent sore throat.
B. Drug history.
C. History of malaria or tuberculosis.
D. History of hepatitis.
E. HIV+.
F. History of diabetes.
G. History of congestive heart failure.

[A. This patient has nephrotic syndrome. Post-infectious GN soon after a sore throat produces nephritic urine. IV drug use and AIDS are associated with focal sclerosis, and skin-popping can cause amyloid nephropathy. Malaria: membranous nephropathy. TB: amyloid.]

21b) What lab tests do not need to be done at this time:
A. CBC, electrolytes, chemistry panel.
B. 24-hour urine protein and creatinine clearance.
C. ANA.
D. Serum complement levels.
E. VDRL.
F. HIV screening.
F. HBsAg.
G. Renal biopsy.

[G. All of the tests should be performed except a renal biopsy. If indicated by these initial tests, a renal biopsy is done. Know these tests!]

21c) All the above lab tests (except renal biopsy) are normal. What is the most likely diagnosis?

A. Post-infectious GN (PIGN).
B. IgA nephropathy.
C. RPGN.
D. Membranoproliferative GN.
E. Minimal change disease.
F. Membranous nephropathy.
G. Amyloid nephropathy.

[F. Membranous nephropathy has been the most common cause of non-diabetic nephrotic syndrome in adults. Now focal sclerosis is proportionally increasing (notice that it is not one of the answer options!). If the patient was in his early 20s or younger, minimal change disease would also be likely. The question says nothing of drug abuse or previous infections so we can, at this point, assume there is no such history.]

22a) An 18-year-old woman is referred to you for the workup of microscopic hematuria found during a school physical. Urine analysis shows: 1+ protein, 2+ blood, 10–20 RBC/HPF, 5 WBC/HPF, 2–5 RBC casts/LPF.

What history is not important in this case?
A. Drug abuse.
B. Recent sore throat or other infection.
C. Recent pulmonary problems.
D. Recent travel outside of the country.
E. Is the patient diabetic.
F. All of the above are important.

[F. This patient has a nephritic syndrome as shown by the WBCs, RBCs, and RBC casts in the urine. All of the history is important: IV drug abuse can cause endocarditis and secondary PIGN. Strep and viral infections: PIGN. Patients with diabetes get nephrotic urine, not nephritic. However, it is still important to know the patient's baseline renal status, so this is important.]

22b) Which one of the following tests does not need to be included in the initial workup?
A. Serum complement levels.
B. ANA.
C. 24-hour urine protein and creatinine clearance.
D. Fractional excretion of sodium.

[D. This patient clearly has a nephritic syndrome. The FE_{Na} is always < 1 in these cases. The serum complement level rules out PIGN, lupus nephritis, and most cases of membranoproliferative GN. ANA is also positive in most (97%) of SLE patients. You do need to quantify the amount of proteinuria and kidney function.]

22c) If the initial tests (from above) are normal, what is the probable cause of this person's renal problem?

A. PIGN.
B. Membranous nephropathy.
C. IgA nephropathy.
D. Focal sclerosis.
E. Lupus nephropathy.

[C. PIGN is ruled out by the normal complement level. The majority of patients with membranoproliferative GN have low complement (but not all). Focal sclerosis and membranous nephropathy are nephrotic only. By process of elimination, the most probable cause is IgA nephropathy.]

OPEN-ENDED QUESTIONS

23) What drugs increase serum creatinine lab results?

[Acetone, cefoxitin, cimetidine, probenecid, and trimethoprim.]

24) Creatinine clearance is the usual way to determine GFR. What effect do the drugs in the above answer, which increase serum creatinine, have on creatinine clearance? What effect do they have on actual GFR?

[Although these drugs either interfere with the creatinine test or decrease creatinine clearance, they have no effect on actual GFR.]

25) The fractional excretion of sodium (FE_{Na}) is the best test for differentiating between what types of renal failure? Give the equation for fractional excretion of sodium.

[$FE_{Na} = Na_{(U/P)}/Cr_{(U/P)}$ x 100. This is the best test for differentiating acute GN and prerenal azotemia from other causes of renal failure. In these 2 cases, the FE_{Na} is normal (< 1%).]

26) What causes the diffuse paresthesias seen in an acute hyperventilation episode?

[Decreased ionized calcium caused by alkalemia.]

27) What are the causes of normal anion gap acidosis and high anion gap acidosis?

[Normal anion gap acidosis (or "hyperchloremic" acidosis) occurs from either a loss of HCO_3^- via the kidney (RTA) or GI tract or from an increase in Cl^- containing acid such as ammonium chloride. The normal anion-gap acidoses are further divided into hypokalemic (usually GI or renal loss) and normo-/hyperkalemic (decreased aldosterone). The most common causes of high anion gap acidosis are ketoacidosis (diabetic, alcoholic, starvation), lactic acidosis, uremia, salicylates, ethylene glycol (makes glycolic and oxalic acid), and methanol (makes formic acid).]

28) Looking at the lytes, BUN, CR, and glucose of a patient, you notice a low HCO_3^-. How can you tell at a glance whether this is a high anion gap acidosis or normal anion gap acidosis?

[If there is no increase in Cl^- equal to the decrease in HCO_3^-, it is a high anion gap acidosis.]

29) Do patients with DKA always present with a high anion gap acidosis?

[Half of diabetics present without volume depletion and have a normal anion gap acidosis.]

30) What do you check for in the urine in a patient with suspected ethylene glycol poisoning?

[Oxalate crystals; these are bipyramidal.]

31) What is the quickest way to determine osmolality if the BUN and glucose are normal?

[Just look at the Na^+ concentration; if it is elevated, osmolality is high.]

32) Hyponatremia is the most common electrolyte abnormality. What is the mechanism for hypertonic hyponatremia?

[Hypertonic hyponatremia is usually caused by hyperglycemia. Glucose causes an osmotic shift of water out of the cells—diluting the serum sodium. Mannitol has the same effect.]

33) Hypotonic hyponatremia is further divided into low, high, and normal volume. In which of these states can total body sodium actually be higher than normal?

[In the high-volume edematous state, in which the patient has retained water and Na^+, but more water than Na^+.]

34) What is the usual cause of normal-volume hypotonic hyponatremia? What drugs can cause this condition?

[SIADH, which can be caused by chlorpropamide, phenothiazines, cyclophosphamide, clofibrate, and vincristine. Diuretics can also cause normal-volume hypotonic hyponatremia if there is sufficient free water replacement.]

35) SIADH is often treated with fluid restriction. What drug may also be useful in certain cases? What are the side effects of this drug?

[Demeclocycline. Photosensitivity; nephrotoxicity in hypoalbuminemic patients.]

36) In a severely hyponatremic patient, what is the possible severe consequence if sodium is replenished too quickly?

[Osmotic demyelination syndrome—also called central pontine myelinolysis.]

37) What potentially serious consequences may occur when a patient gets too rapid a correction of a hyperosmotic state?

[Cellular swelling.]

38) How do you calculate the amount of free water needed in a patient with hypernatremia?

[$Volume_{water}$ = .6(body weight in kg)(Na^+_{serum} - 145)/145]

39) How do you differentiate central from nephrogenic diabetes insipidus?

[Water-restriction test. With central DI undergoing water restriction, the ADH remains low and the urine unconcentrated. With nephrogenic DI, the urine is again unconcentrated, although the ADH is appropriately elevated.]

40) What can be used to treat mild cases of DI?

[Chlorpropamide and thiazide diuretics can be used to treat mild cases of central DI. Nephrogenic DI is treated with thiazide diuretics.]

41) How do thiazides and loop diuretics differ in their handling of calcium?

[Loop diuretics increase calcium excretion, whereas thiazide diuretics decrease calcium excretion.]

42) In the distal tubule where sodium is actively resorbed, how are potassium and H^+ excreted? How does a metabolic acidosis or alkalosis affect this excretion?

[K^+ and H^+ are excreted along the electrical gradient caused by the active resorption of Na^+. H^+ and K^+ compete for excretion along this gradient. If the patient is acidotic (high H^+), more H^+ than K^+ will be excreted, and the patient will tend to have hyperkalemia. If the patient is hyperkalemic, the patient will tend to be acidotic for the same reason.]

43) Why is spironolactone potassium-sparing? How can it cause acidosis?

[Spironolactone is an aldosterone antagonist. This prevents the formation of the electrical gradient along which K^+ and H^+ are excreted. This makes the diuretic potassium-sparing and causes a tendency for the development of metabolic acidosis.]

44) What drugs should you not give to a patient who has hyperkalemia due to a hyporeninemic hypoaldosteronism?

[NSAIDs, ACE inhibitors, beta-blockers, and heparin.]

45) What is the treatment for severe hyperkalemia with ECG changes? Know the reason these drugs are given, onset of action, and duration of action for each.

[Treatment utilizes IV calcium, insulin and glucose, $NaHCO_3$, and K^+ binding resins. Immediate treatment is IV calcium: either 1 amp calcium chloride or 3 amps of calcium gluconate. Within 5 minutes, IV calcium counters the effect of the high K^+ on the heart. Then give insulin and glucose, which increase entry of K^+ into cells—onset is 15–30 minutes, duration 12–24 hours. Then give $NaHCO_3$ (shifts K^+ into the cells—onset in 15–45 minutes, duration 12–24 hours), and K^+ binding resins, which work more slowly. Remember: The hyperkalemic ECG changes are peaked T waves, widened QRS, and severe arrhythmias.]

46) Name the common causes of hypokalemia.

[Gastrointestinal K^+ loss (diarrhea, fistulas, and laxatives), renal K^+ wasting (hyperaldosteronism or gentamicin), alkalosis, exogenous insulin, IV glucose administration or high insulin production, and hypomagnesemia.]

47) What is the most common cause of normotensive hypokalemia? What should you suspect in the normotensive hypokalemic patient with a hyperchloremic acidosis?

[Diuretics. Type 1 RTA.]

48) Name 3 secondary effects of hypokalemia.

[U waves on the ECG, decreased deep tendon reflexes, and occasionally rhabdomyolysis.]

49) How much does total calcium decrease for each decrease in albumin of 1?

[0.7.]

50) How does rhabdomyolysis affect serum calcium levels?

[Rhabdomyolysis can cause hypocalcemia.]

51) How is severe hypermagnesemia treated?

[IV calcium +/- dialysis.]

52) Name 4 drugs that commonly cause hypomagnesemia.

[Amphotericin B, diuretics, gentamicin, and cisplatin.]

53) Why must magnesium occasionally be given to the patient with hypocalcemia or hypokalemia?

[Because hypomagnesemia itself can cause hypocalcemia and hypokalemia.]

54) In what way are refractory cardiac arrhythmias associated with magnesium?

[Refractory cardiac rhythms appear to be associated not only with hypomagnesemia, but also with depleted magnesium stores—even with normal serum levels!]

55) If an alcoholic patient presents for detox, and several days later becomes extremely weak, what chemistry should you check?

[Serum phosphate level. This may be normal on admission and only decrease as the glycogen level is returned to normal after a normal diet is reestablished.]

56) 95% of all hypertension is primary. Is mortality and morbidity higher for women vs. men? For blacks vs. whites?

[Mortality and morbidity : men > women; blacks > whites.]

57) If a young patient presents with obesity and mild hypertension, what lab test should you do?

[Cholesterol level.]

58) In what way might hyperinsulinemia be a cause of primary hypertension?

[Hyperinsulinemia can (theoretically, at least) cause volume retention, vascular hypertrophy, and sympathetic overactivity which, in turn, causes HTN.]

59) If an otherwise healthy patient presents for a job physical and is found to have a diastolic blood pressure of 92, when would you recheck it?

[Recheck blood pressure within 2 months.]

60) What is the standard workup for newly diagnosed hypertension?

[Per the JNC 7: Initial lab tests for all hypertensive patients: CBC, serum chemistry (K^+, Na^+, creatinine, fasting glucose, total cholesterol, HDL cholesterol), and a 12-lead ECG.]

61) Name 6 indications for further evaluation for secondary causes of hypertension.

[Abrupt onset, age < 30 years, stage III HTN, refractory HTN, hypercalcemia, hypokalemia with kaliuresis, systolic-diastolic bruits in the epigastrium or lateralizing over a kidney (systolic bruits alone are not an indication.)]

62) What are the 2 main causes of renovascular hypertension? Which age group tends to get which cause?

[Onset < 30 years old: fibromuscular dysplasia. Onset > 50 years old: renal artery atherosclerosis.]

63) What type of abdominal bruit suggests renovascular hypertension?

[A bruit with both systolic and diastolic components.]

64) How do you screen for renovascular hypertension? How is it confirmed?

[Captopril test. Renal artery arteriography.]

65) What are the risk factors for pregnancy-induced hypertension (preeclampsia)?

[Serum creatinine > 1.2, blood pressure > 160/100, increased liver enzymes, retinal hemorrhage, platelet count < 100,000, and microangiopathic hemolytic anemia.]

66) If a pregnant patient develops hypertension in the second trimester, what is the probable etiology?

[Essential hypertension. Pregnancy-induced hypertension occurs only in the 3rd trimester.]

67) Why should patients with bilateral renal artery obstruction or severe CHF be watched carefully when on ACE inhibitors?

[Because renal function becomes angiotensin II-dependent in these patients, and ACEI/ARBs can cause GFR to decrease and worsen.]

68) In initiating therapy in a patient with hypertension, the drug of choice may vary, depending on various factors. Which are the drugs of choice for patients with ischemic heart disease? If the patient has LVH? If the patient has CHF?

[Ischemic heart disease: Calcium-channel blockers or beta-blockers. LVH: ACE inhibitors, and calcium-channel blockers. CHF: ACE inhibitors or diuretics (but watch for worsening azotemia.)]

69) When are beta-blockers usually avoided?

[CHF, reactive airway disease, hyperlipidemia, and PVD.]

70) What causes the retinopathy in malignant hypertension?

[Retinal artery spasm.]

71) What is the treatment for malignant hypertension?

[Initially decrease the BP by 25%. This is done within minutes to 2 hours. Then toward 160/100 mmHg within 2–6 hours. Drugs used have a rapid onset of action and usually can be oral: loop diuretics, beta-blockers, alpha$_2$-antagonists, or calcium antagonists. Do not use sublingual nifedipine! Too many problems with serious side effects.]

72) Why are nitrates not used to treat hypertension in the patient with severe LVH?

[These patients have a diastolic dysfunction, which is worsened by preload reducers. Negative inotropics, such as beta-blockers or calcium-channel blockers, are the initial drugs of choice. Diuretics can be used with care.]

73) Name the drugs that are associated with prerenal failure.

[Diuretics, NSAIDs, ACE inhibitors, and interleukin-2.]

74) To what type of renal failure is the patient who is severely hypoalbuminemic most susceptible?

[Prerenal failure.]

75) In what types of renal problems is the $FE_{Na} < 1\%$?

[Prerenal azotemia and acute GN.]

76) What is the usual cause of postrenal failure?

[Bladder outlet obstruction.]

77) Of the 4 causes of intrarenal failure (GNs, acute interstitial nephritis, vascular problems, and ATN), which is the most common?

[ATN.]

78) The most common cause of ATN is renal hypoperfusion. What most commonly causes this hypoperfusion?

[Surgery.]

79) What are other causes of ATN?

[Myoglobinuria, heavy metals, hypercalcemia, hemoglobinuria, contrast dye, and drugs—especially aminoglycosides, amphotericin B, methotrexate, and cisplatin.]

80) How is ATN diagnosed?

[Clinical setting, muddy brown casts on reanalysis, and urine osmolality < 400, Urine Na is > 20, and $FE_{Na} \gg 1\%$.]

81) What type of ATN does gentamicin usually cause? Is this more or less likely to resolve?

[Nonoliguric ATN. More likely to resolve.]

82) What are the symptoms of multiple cholesterol emboli syndrome (MCES)? How is this diagnosed?

[Stepwise deterioration in renal function after a diagnostic catheterization. Skin biopsy is diagnostic.]

83) If a patient with ATN has hypocalcemia, hyperphosphatemia, high uric acid, and a very high creatinine with a low BUN/creatinine ratio, what is the most probable cause of the ATN?

[Rhabdomyolysis.]

84) How low a potassium level do you expect in a patient with hypokalemic-induced rhabdomyolysis?

[It may be normal!]

85) Explain how each of the following chemotherapies can cause ARF: methotrexate, cisplatin, mitomycin C, antimetabolites.

[Methotrexate: precipitates and obstructs the tubules; cisplatin: directly nephrotoxic; mitomycin C: hemolytic uremic syndrome; antimetabolites: uric acid nephropathy.]

86) What is the usual cause of most GNs?

[Antigen-antibody (immune complex) reaction.]

87) What are 2 classic findings in the urine in nephrotic syndrome?

[Heavy proteinuria and urine fat. The protein is > 2.5–3.5 gm/dl or 50 mg/kg/d.]

88) Why do patients with nephrotic syndrome tend to get infections with *H. flu* and *Strep pneumoniae*?

[The protein lost through the glomeruli includes gamma globulins, which protect against encapsulated entities.]

89) Why do patients with nephrotic syndrome tend to get renal vein thrombosis and pulmonary emboli?

[They become hypercoagulable due to loss of antithrombin III.]

90) How does urine sediment differ between nephrotic and nephritic syndrome?

[Nephritic syndrome has "active" urine sediment. This consists of dysmorphic RBCs and WBCs, and RBC, WBC, and granular casts. Nephrotic syndrome: presents primarily with heavy proteinuria and urine fat ("oval fat bodies").]

91) If a patient with a history of pneumonia several weeks prior to admission presents with new-onset proteinuria with RBC casts, what is the most likely cause?

[Post-infectious GN.]

92) What is the treatment for post-infectious GN?

[Antibiotics.]

93) What is the location and morphology of the immune complex deposits in post-infectious GN?

[Subepithelial glomerular humps.]

94) What is the most common type of GN?

[IgA nephropathy (Mesangial proliferative GN).]

95) What type of nephropathy does Buerger disease or Henoch-Schönlein purpura cause?

[IgA nephropathy (Mesangial proliferative GN).]

96) If a male patient presents with gross hematuria and mild proteinuria after exercising, what GN would you suspect?

[IgA nephropathy (Mesangial proliferative GN).]

97) What are the immunoglobulins involved with mesangial proliferative GN?

[Usually IgA, but occasionally IgM.]

98) What type of GN usually presents with acute, severe renal failure? What are the causes of it?

[RPGN; vasculitis (polyarteritis nodosa and Wegener granulomatosis), SLE, and Goodpasture syndrome. Other GNs occasionally evolve into RPGN.]

99) What are the different implications of cellular crescents vs. fibrous crescents on a kidney biopsy?

[Cellular crescents are caused by an acute inflammatory process, which may be reversible. Fibrous crescents indicate scarring and an irreversible condition.]

100) What 2 antibody tests are used in the diagnosis of rapidly progressive GN?

[Anti-GBM (anti-glomerular basement membrane) antibody is checked first for the possibility of Goodpasture syndrome. If it is negative, check the ANCA (anti-neutrophil cytoplasmic autoantibodies).]

101) If a patient presents with acute, severe renal failure and the anti-GBM antibodies are negative, but there are high titers of ANCA antibodies, what are 3 possible causes?

[Wegener's, polyarteritis nodosa, or idiopathic crescentic GN. Wegener's is usually c-ANCA positive, while the latter 2 can be positive for either p- or c-ANCA.]

102) What type of GN is associated with SLE?

[SLE can cause just about any type of GN.]

103) What type of GN has a double-layered–looking membrane on electron microscopy?

[Membranoproliferative GN.]

104) Lupus nephritis, post-infectious nephritis, and membranoproliferative nephritis all have associative hypocomplementemia. How do the changes over time in the level of C3 aid in the differential diagnosis between membranoproliferative and PIGN?

[The C3 in post-infectious GN stays low for < 3 months, while it stays low indefinitely in membranoproliferative GN.]

105) What is the most common cause of nephrotic syndrome in children? How is it diagnosed? How is it treated?

[Minimal change disease. Diagnose by electron microscopy (fusion of the epithelial cell foot processes) and examination of the urine sediment ("Maltese crosses"). Treat with corticosteroids first, then cyclophosphamide or cyclosporine.]

106) What are the 2 most common causes of nephrotic syndrome in non-diabetic adults?

[Membranous nephropathy and focal sclerosis.]

107) What nephropathy do you expect in a patient with a solid tumor, who then develops nephrotic syndrome?

[Membranous nephropathy.]

108) Which patient groups with membranous nephropathy have a much better prognosis?

[Women and children. Note that membranous glomerulonephropathy is very rare in children.]

109) What decreases the rate of decline in renal function in diabetic nephropathy?

[Good control of hypertension and glucose level and use of an ACE inhibitor or ARB; a low-protein diet may also help.]

110) What type of RTA is associated with diabetic nephropathy?

[Diabetic nephropathy is associated with Type 4 RTA.]

111) What is the differential diagnosis of a renal biopsy showing very large hyaline-appearing masses in the glomerulus? How are these 2 entities differentiated?

[Diabetic vs. light chain nephropathy. Besides history, the congo red stain of amyloid has a unique "apple-green birefringence."]

112) What is the cause of amyloid nephropathy in chronic drug abusers? What type of amyloid is seen in these patients?

[Chronic skin infections from "skin-popping." "AA" type.]

113) What type of kidney malfunction do heavy metals usually cause?

[Chronic interstitial nephritis. They can also cause ATN and Type 2 RTA.]

114) What is the significance of having glucose in the urine yet a normal serum glucose?

[This is seen with chronic interstitial nephritis, Type 2 RTA, and pregnancy. Need more tests!]

115) What is the protein level in the urine of a patient with NSAID-induced chronic interstitial nephritis?

[In contrast to the other types of chronic interstitial nephritis, NSAIDs cause nephrotic-range proteinuria.]

116) If a patient presents with microcytic anemia, CKD, and gout, what entity must be ruled out?

[Lead nephropathy.]

117) How is renal osteodystrophy caused? Why should aluminum be used sparingly in patients with this problem?

[This is a hyperparathyroid bone disease caused by both decreased conversion of $1(OH)D_3$ to $1,25\text{-}(OH)_2D_3$ by the defective kidneys and high serum phosphate from decreased renal excretion. Aluminum can exacerbate this problem and actually cause aluminum-induced osteomalacia.]

118) What are the most common causes of death in chronic kidney disease?

[Most common causes of death in CKD: Cardiovascular problems; then infection.]

119) When is dialysis started in chronic kidney disease?

[When the CKD patient starts experiencing uremic symptoms and CrCl < 5–10 μl/min.]

120) What problems can aluminum accumulation cause in chronic kidney disease?

[Weakness, anemia, encephalopathy (dialysis dementia), and a vitamin D-resistant osteomalacia. This is usually due to aluminum-containing antacids.]

121) What is the main complication in CAPD? How is this treated?

[Peritonitis. This is usually successfully treated with outpatient intraperitoneal antibiotics.]

122) What type of renal diseases do not recur after a renal transplant?

[Post-infectious GN and interstitial nephritis do not recur after a renal transplant. Renal diseases that do recur after transplant include rapidly progressive GN, mesangial (IgA, Berger), membranoproliferative GN, and idiopathic focal/segmental sclerosis.]

123) Does dialysis or renal transplant reverse the motor neuropathy that diabetics get? The sensory neuropathy?

[Both dialysis and renal transplant reverse the platelet dysfunction, renal osteodystrophy, and sensory and cognitive dysfunction. Only transplant can reverse the late manifestations of small-vessel calcification and motor neuropathy.]

124) What anti-gout medicine is ineffective in CKD?

[Probenecid; it usually works by increasing the renal excretion of uric acid.]

125) What does Alport syndrome (hereditary nephritis) have in common with Goodpasture syndrome?

[Both affect the basement membrane.]

126) If a female patient presents with microscopic hematuria and has a history of male relatives dying of renal failure, what is the probable diagnosis?

[Alport syndrome.]

127) When do you need to screen for cerebral aneurysms in patients with polycystic kidney disease?

[When the patient is symptomatic or when there is a family history suggestive of cerebral aneurysms.]

128) What type of antibiotics are used for kidney infections in patients with polycystic kidney disease? Why?

[Use lipid-soluble antibiotics, such as quinolones, trimethoprim, erythromycin, chloramphenicol, tetracycline, and clindamycin, in patients with kidney infection and polycystic kidney disease because they penetrate better.]

129) What are the most common types of kidney stones?

[Calcium.]

130) What is the workup after the initial kidney stone?

[Workup following initial stone passage usually includes chemical analysis of the stone, calcium level (to rule out a hyperparathyroidism problem), electrolytes (to rule out Type 1 distal RTA), U/A with C+S, and IVP.]

131) How does citrate inhibit calcium stone formation?

[Citrate chelates calcium.]

132) What are 2 oxalate precursors that may cause renal stones?

[Vitamin C and ethylene glycol.]

133) What conditions predispose to uric acid stones?

[High serum uric acid and acidic urine. Myeloproliferative syndromes, chemotherapy, and Lesch-Nyhan syndrome can cause hyperuricosuria.]

134) What type of stones do you think of when you see staghorn calculi on the abdominal x-ray?

[Struvite stones.]